MW01170916

THE PEPTIDE PROTOCOLS MASTER BIBLE

Evidence-Based Guide Made Simple to Next-Generation Peptides & Combos | Usage, Dosing & Cycling for Weight Loss, Muscle Growth, Longevity & Body Optimization

Dr. Christopher J. Calloway

TABLE OF CONTENTS

BOOK 1

1

INTRODUCTION TO PEPTIDES SCIENCE

What are Peptides?

Peptides have become an increasingly important area of focus in health and wellness, but what exactly are they, and why are they so impactful?

Peptides are essentially short sequences of amino acids, the fundamental components that make up proteins. These smaller chains are created when amino acids link together in specific arrangements, making peptides unique in their structure and function compared to full proteins.

While proteins are typically made up of hundreds of amino acids, peptides are generally smaller, containing anywhere from two to about fifty amino acids linked together in a specific sequence. Despite their simplicity, these small molecules play essential roles in almost every biological function, acting as messengers, signaling molecules, and catalysts for various processes throughout the body.

Understanding peptides begins with understanding the role of amino acids, the molecules that make up proteins and peptides alike. There are 20 amino acids in the human body, each with distinct properties and functions. When linked together in different sequences and lengths, they form chains that can influence nearly every function, from muscle growth to immune response and cognitive processing. Think of peptides as the "words" formed by amino acids, where each unique sequence sends a particular message or performs a unique function. This targeted action gives peptides their extraordinary versatility and effectiveness in promoting various health benefits.

Why Peptides Are Unique

One of the defining features of peptides is their specificity. While many treatments or supplements aim to improve health broadly, peptides act in very targeted ways, binding to specific cell receptors and triggering precise responses in the body. For example, certain peptides bind to receptors in the pituitary gland, which then releases growth hormone, a critical factor in cell regeneration, muscle growth, and fat metabolism. Other peptides can influence the brain, promoting neurotransmitter release, which affects memory, mood, and focus.

This specificity makes peptides incredibly efficient; they act on the body's cells in a targeted manner, often with fewer side effects than broader, less specific treatments. Peptides have a "bioactive" nature, meaning that they can alter biological processes and actively work within the body to influence particular functions. Because they are naturally occurring and often identical to the body's own peptides, these molecules are generally well-tolerated and are often metabolized quickly, reducing the risk of adverse reactions.

Classification of Peptides by Size

Peptides can be classified based on the number of amino acids they contain, reflecting their structural and functional diversity. This classification is not only foundational in biochemistry but also crucial in determining the biological roles and applications of peptides in therapeutic, diagnostic, and industrial settings.

1. Oligopeptides (2–10 Amino Acids)

Short chains composed of fewer than 10 amino acids.

- **Examples**:
  - **Dipeptides**: Contain two amino acids (e.g., aspartame, a dipeptide used as an artificial sweetener).
  - **Tripeptides**: Composed of three amino acids (e.g., glutathione, critical in cellular redox balance).
  - **Tetrapeptides and Pentapeptides**: Extend biological functions like signaling (e.g., tuftsin, a tetrapeptide involved in immune modulation).
- **Characteristics**:
  - Highly soluble in water.
  - Rapidly absorbed and metabolized.
  - Often used in cosmetic formulations for skin repair and rejuvenation (e.g., collagen peptides).
- **Applications**: Nutraceuticals, cosmetics, and as intermediates in larger protein synthesis.

2. Polypeptides (11–50 Amino Acids)

Chains with 11 to 50 amino acids, forming a bridge between small oligopeptides and full proteins.

- **Examples**:
  - **Insulin**: A 51-amino acid polypeptide critical for glucose metabolism.
  - **Amyloid Beta**: A 42-amino acid polypeptide linked to Alzheimer's disease pathology.
- **Characteristics**:
  - Display secondary structures such as alpha-helices or beta-sheets.
  - Can act as hormones, enzymes, or structural molecules.
- **Applications**: Therapeutics, such as hormone replacement therapy (e.g., synthetic insulin) and neuropeptide research.

3. Proteins (>50 Amino Acids)

- While not classified strictly as peptides, chains longer than 50 amino acids are generally considered proteins.
- Overlap exists in classification, as some long polypeptides exhibit peptide-like properties depending on their function and structure.

Specialized Size-Based Classifications

1. **Micropeptides (Less than 100 Amino Acids)**:
   - Derived from larger coding and non-coding RNA.
   - Play roles in gene regulation and cellular processes.
   - Examples: Myoregulin, a micropeptide that regulates muscle function.
2. **Macrocyclic Peptides**:
   - Feature cyclic structures that improve stability and membrane permeability.
   - Applications include drug development for challenging targets.
   - Example: Cyclosporin, an immunosuppressive cyclic peptide.
3. **Mini-Proteins**:
   - Include small proteins with highly conserved sequences and compact structures.
   - Function in diverse biological systems, from enzymatic activity to signaling.

Relevance of Peptide Size in Applications

Therapeutics:

- Smaller peptides are easier to synthesize and administer but often have limited stability.
- Larger peptides or polypeptides have more complex biological activities but face challenges in delivery and stability.

Diagnostics: Short peptides can serve as biomarkers or probes for specific diseases.

Material Science: Peptide size influences mechanical properties when used in hydrogels or nanomaterials.

Challenges in Size-Based Peptide Research

- Stability issues for smaller peptides due to enzymatic degradation.
- Higher complexity of synthesis for longer polypeptides.
- Regulatory hurdles for novel peptides in clinical applications.

Bioactive Properties of Peptides

Peptides are involved in almost every physiological process, and they are essential for maintaining balance and function in the body. Below are just a few examples of their varied roles:

Hormone Regulation: Many peptides act as hormones, carrying messages between organs and tissues to regulate essential functions. For instance, insulin is a peptide hormone that regulates blood glucose levels, while oxytocin, another peptide hormone, is involved in bonding and emotional responses.

Immune System Modulation: Some peptides help regulate immune function, enhancing the body's response to pathogens and injury. Some peptides promote the production of white blood cells, which are essential for enhancing the immune system and combating infections.

Muscle and Tissue Repair: Growth hormone-releasing peptides (GHRPs) and other muscle-focused peptides stimulate tissue repair and muscle growth, making them popular in fitness and physical rehabilitation.

Cognitive Support: Certain peptides interact with brain receptors to improve memory, focus, and cognitive resilience. These neuropeptides play roles in learning, mood regulation, and even sleep.

Skin and Cosmetic Benefits: Peptides like collagen-stimulating peptides have become popular in skincare due to their ability to promote elasticity and reduce signs of aging by stimulating collagen production, which can keep skin firm and resilient.

How Peptides Differ from Other Treatments

While other treatments—like pharmaceutical drugs or even traditional supplements—might broadly target health issues, peptides offer a unique advantage in their capacity to work with the body's natural signaling processes. Traditional pharmaceuticals often interact with a broad spectrum of biological pathways, which can lead to side effects as they don't always discriminate between desirable and undesirable targets. Peptides, by contrast, are like keys to specific locks; they fit perfectly with certain receptors, which allows them to exert a particular effect with a high degree of precision. This focused approach reduces the potential for unintended consequences, making peptides an appealing option for those who seek targeted interventions.

The Evolution of Peptide Therapeutics

While peptides have been recognized in scientific circles for over a century, their application as therapeutic agents has only recently come to the forefront, thanks in large part to advances in biotechnology. Peptides were once difficult and costly to manufacture, but modern synthetic techniques now allow for large-scale production, making them accessible for both medical and research applications. These advancements have spurred a significant interest in peptide-based therapies, leading to an explosion of research into their potential uses across many fields, including endocrinology, neurology, and dermatology.

Today, peptides are not only used in clinical settings but are also gaining popularity in areas like anti-aging, athletic performance, and cognitive health. The increase in knowledge about peptides has also led to safer, more effective delivery methods, such as injectable peptides, topical applications, and even orally stable forms. As understanding deepens, the list of peptides available for specific health benefits continues to grow, allowing practitioners and enthusiasts alike to explore the diverse potential of these molecules in optimizing health and wellness.

The Science Behind Peptide Signaling

Peptide signaling represents a fundamental mechanism of molecular communication in biological systems, playing a pivotal role in processes such as growth, metabolism, immune response, and neural activity. Below is a detailed analysis of the concepts central to peptide signaling, encompassing its molecular underpinnings, pathways, and therapeutic implications.

What Is Peptide Signaling?

Peptide signaling refers to the process by which peptide molecules serve as signaling agents, binding to specific receptors on target cells to elicit biological responses. Peptides function as hormones, neurotransmitters, or cytokines, facilitating communication between cells, tissues, and organs. This signaling is crucial for maintaining homeostasis and coordinating complex physiological processes.

Molecular Communication

At the heart of peptide signaling lies molecular communication—a process that relies on the synthesis, secretion, and detection of signaling peptides. These molecules are produced in the cell and released into the extracellular space or bloodstream. Target cells detect these peptides through highly specific receptors, initiating a cascade of molecular events that convert extracellular signals into cellular responses.

- **Specificity:** The ability of peptides to target specific receptors ensures precision in signaling, minimizing unintended effects.
- **Dynamic Range:** Peptides operate across various concentration ranges, allowing nuanced regulation of biological processes.

Receptor-Mediated Signaling

Peptide signaling is mediated by interactions with membrane-bound receptors, typically part of the G protein-coupled receptor (GPCR) family or receptor tyrosine kinases (RTKs). These receptors are designed to recognize peptide ligands with high specificity and affinity.

- **GPCRs:** Many peptide hormones, such as glucagon and oxytocin, bind to GPCRs, triggering intracellular signaling cascades via second messengers like cAMP or calcium ions.

- **RTKs:** Insulin and other growth-related peptides activate RTKs, which phosphorylate intracellular proteins to initiate transcriptional changes.

The receptor-peptide binding event induces conformational changes in the receptor, enabling it to interact with downstream signaling molecules.

Signal Transduction Pathways

Signal transduction refers to the series of molecular events that transmit the signal from a receptor on the cell's surface to intracellular targets. This typically involves a series of proteins that amplify and propagate the signal, culminating in specific cellular responses.

Key pathways in peptide signaling include:

1. **cAMP Pathway:** Common in GPCR-mediated signaling, this pathway uses cyclic AMP as a secondary messenger to activate protein kinase A (PKA), affecting gene expression and enzyme activity.
2. **MAPK Pathway:** Activated by RTKs, the mitogen-activated protein kinase (MAPK) pathway regulates cell division, differentiation, and survival.
3. **PI3K-AKT Pathway:** Often involved in metabolic and growth-related signaling, this pathway mediates responses to insulin and other peptides.

Biological Response Networks

Peptide signaling orchestrates intricate biological response networks that integrate multiple signaling inputs to generate coordinated cellular behaviors. These networks are characterized by feedback loops, cross-talk between pathways, and signal amplification.

- **Feedback Mechanisms:** Negative feedback ensures signal termination, while positive feedback can sustain or amplify responses.
- **Cross-Talk:** Interactions between signaling pathways allow cells to fine-tune responses and adapt to environmental changes.
- **Temporal Dynamics:** The timing and duration of peptide signals influence outcomes, such as transient vs. sustained activation of pathways.

Therapeutic Implications

Peptide signaling pathways are critical targets for therapeutic intervention. Dysregulation of these pathways is implicated in numerous diseases, including cancer, diabetes, cardiovascular conditions, and autoimmune disorders. Advances in peptide-based therapies harness the specificity and potency of peptides to restore or modulate signaling.

- **Peptide Drugs:** Therapeutic peptides, such as GLP-1 analogs for diabetes, mimic or enhance natural peptide signaling.
- **Antagonists and Inhibitors:** Molecules that block peptide receptors or signaling components can inhibit overactive pathways, as seen in cancer treatment.
- **Delivery Systems:** Innovations in peptide drug delivery, such as nanoparticle carriers, improve stability and targeting.

What is Meant by "PEPTIDE PROTOCOLS"?

"Peptide protocols" refer to structured, scientifically-informed guidelines for using peptides to achieve specific health or performance outcomes. These protocols typically include details about which peptides to use, optimal dosages, timing, cycling, and potential combinations to maximize their effectiveness while minimizing risks.

Peptide protocols are crafted with several key considerations in mind:

- **Selection of Peptides**

The choice of peptide(s) is the foundation of any protocol, as each peptide has a unique action. For instance, some peptides stimulate growth hormone production, while others target inflammation, muscle repair, or cognitive processes. Selecting the appropriate peptides requires a deep understanding of how each molecule interacts with the body's systems. A peptide protocol might use a single peptide or a combination, known as a "stack," which leverages the synergistic effects of multiple peptides working together.

- **Dosage and Administration**

Proper dosing is essential in peptide protocols to ensure both safety and effectiveness. Too low of a dose may be ineffective, while too high a dose can cause undesirable side effects. Protocols often specify initial dosages, as well as incremental increases (called titration) to help the body acclimate. Additionally, protocols will outline the best method of administration—whether by injection, oral intake, or topical application—as peptides vary in their absorption and stability based on the delivery route.

- **Timing and Cycling**

Peptides can produce powerful effects, but they work best when used cyclically. Cycling means using the peptide for a specific period, such as several weeks, followed by a rest period, or "off-cycle." This on-and-off approach prevents desensitization, where the body becomes accustomed to the peptide and diminishes its response. Cycling also helps to reduce any potential long-term side effects and allows the body's natural functions to remain balanced. Timing considerations include daily schedules (e.g., morning vs. evening doses) and whether the peptide should be taken on an empty stomach or alongside other compounds.

- **Combining Peptides (Peptide Stacks)**

A protocol might include a combination of peptides to achieve multiple goals simultaneously. For instance, a muscle-building protocol might stack growth hormone-releasing peptides with a peptide that reduces muscle soreness, enhancing both growth and recovery. Each peptide in a stack has a complementary role, and understanding how these molecules work together is essential to creating an effective protocol.

- **Monitoring and Adjustment**

Every individual responds differently to peptides due to factors like genetics, lifestyle, and overall health. Monitoring one's response is a critical part of any protocol, allowing for adjustments in dosage, timing, or peptide selection as needed. Protocols encourage users to keep a log of any changes in performance, mood, physical changes, and side effects. This feedback loop ensures that peptide use is adapted to meet each person's unique needs, rather than taking a one-size-fits-all approach.

The Purpose of Peptide Protocols: Structured Use for Targeted Outcomes

The purpose of peptide protocols is to take a methodical approach that enhances the benefits of peptides while minimizing potential risks. Because peptides can have potent effects on the body, especially when dealing with hormones or neuropeptides, it's important to follow protocols developed from both scientific research and clinical experience. Protocols give a roadmap to users, providing clarity on how to harness peptides safely and effectively for their specific goals.

Examples of Common Peptide Protocols

Each protocol is tailored to a specific purpose, and some examples include:

Fat Loss Protocols: Peptides that stimulate lipolysis (the breakdown of fat cells) are often combined with peptides that increase metabolic rate, helping users lose fat while preserving lean muscle mass.

Muscle-Building Protocols: Growth hormone-releasing peptides or IGF (Insulin-like Growth Factor) peptides are typically used here, often in combination with peptides that reduce inflammation, enhancing muscle repair and building.

Cognitive Enhancement Protocols: Neuropeptides that influence neurotransmitter release can improve focus, memory, and mood, and protocols might include cycling recommendations to prevent dependency.

Anti-Aging and Skin Health Protocols: These protocols focus on peptides that promote collagen production and cellular repair, with guidelines for long-term use to sustain skin elasticity and reduce signs of aging.

The History and Evolution of Peptides

The story of peptides begins in the early 20th century with the exploration of amino acids and proteins, the building blocks of peptides. Over the past century, peptides have evolved from obscure scientific curiosities to some of the most promising therapeutic agents available today, touching areas from endocrinology and neurology to cosmetic dermatology and weight management. Understanding how peptides came to be central in modern medicine, research, and even daily health routines involves an exciting journey through scientific discovery, technological advancement, and medical breakthroughs.

Early Discovery: The Foundation of Peptide Science

The discovery of peptides is intertwined with our understanding of proteins, which are essentially long chains of amino acids. Scientists began studying proteins in the 19th century, intrigued by their presence in tissues and organs. In 1901, the German chemist Emil Fischer made groundbreaking advances in understanding proteins by successfully linking amino acids into chains. This discovery laid the foundation for peptide science, as peptides are shorter chains of amino acids. Fischer's work eventually earned him the Nobel Prize in Chemistry, and his methods became central to peptide and protein research.

One of the first identified peptides, oxytocin, a small hormone that influences childbirth, lactation, and social bonding, was synthesized in the 1950s by chemist Vincent du Vigneaud. Synthesizing oxytocin marked the first time scientists could recreate a peptide in the lab, demonstrating that it was possible to control these small yet powerful molecules. This discovery sparked interest in the potential of peptide synthesis for therapeutic use and opened the door to further exploration.

Peptide Hormones and the Rise of Biotechnology (1960s-1980s)

Peptide research took a major leap forward in the 1960s with the discovery of more peptide hormones, such as insulin, vasopressin, and glucagon. Insulin, a critical hormone for regulating blood sugar, became one of the most important peptides in medical history. By identifying its structure, scientists could produce it artificially, which revolutionized diabetes treatment and saved countless lives. Understanding the biological roles of these peptide hormones deepened scientific interest in how manipulating peptide levels could influence health outcomes.

As the biotechnology industry emerged in the 1970s and 1980s, scientists developed sophisticated methods for synthesizing and modifying peptides. Recombinant DNA technology allowed for the mass production of peptide-based drugs, making them widely available. Biotechnology companies like Genentech were at the forefront of this peptide revolution, producing peptide hormones, such as synthetic human growth hormone (HGH), which was initially developed to treat growth disorders in children. These advances highlighted the therapeutic power of peptides and accelerated peptide drug development.

The Therapeutic Revolution of Peptides (1990s-2000s)

The 1990s saw an explosion of interest in peptides as potential therapies. Advances in understanding the human genome and molecular biology allowed scientists to identify hundreds of peptides with specific functions in the body. This decade also introduced the concept of peptide libraries, which allowed researchers to test thousands of peptides in quick succession, identifying those with specific biological activities. This high-throughput screening approach was instrumental in discovering peptides that could target diseases or enhance physiological functions.

In the 2000s, peptide therapeutics took off as scientists developed stabilization techniques that made peptides more effective in the body. Initially, peptides faced limitations as therapeutics due to their short half-lives and tendency to degrade quickly in the bloodstream. Innovations like peptide pegylation (attaching polyethylene glycol chains to peptides) extended their lifespan, making them more practical for medical use. Modified peptides could now be administered less frequently, improving patient compliance and therapeutic effectiveness.

This era saw the rise of several game-changing peptide drugs. For instance, GLP-1 agonists (glucagon-like peptide-1) became widely used to manage diabetes by enhancing insulin secretion and reducing appetite. Peptide therapeutics for conditions like osteoporosis (e.g., teriparatide, a parathyroid hormone analog) and multiple sclerosis (e.g., glatiramer acetate) also emerged, validating the therapeutic potential of peptides across a wide range of medical disciplines.

Modern Peptides: Targeted Therapies, Precision Medicine, and Beyond

In the past two decades, peptide research has surged forward, propelled by advances in precision medicine, computational biology, and personalized healthcare. Today, peptides are increasingly being designed to target very specific tissues or receptors, reducing side effects and enhancing efficacy. For example, tumor-targeting peptides have been developed that can attach to cancer cells while sparing healthy ones, providing a targeted approach to cancer treatment. By focusing on specific cellular receptors or pathways, these peptides minimize off-target effects and offer a higher therapeutic window.

Peptides are also central to the field of regenerative medicine and anti-aging therapies. Growth hormone secretagogues (like Ipamorelin and MOD-GRF 1-29) and peptides promoting collagen production have found applications in skin care, muscle recovery, and even cognitive enhancement. With applications ranging from fitness and weight management to immune modulation, peptides have become essential tools for improving quality of life and longevity.

Cosmetic and Wellness Applications: Peptides in Daily Life

One fascinating evolution in peptides has been their crossover from clinical to cosmetic and wellness applications. Cosmetic peptides, such as palmitoyl pentapeptide-4 (found in anti-aging skincare), mimic proteins that stimulate collagen production, reducing wrinkles and promoting skin elasticity. Argireline, often called "Botox in a Bottle," is another cosmetic peptide that temporarily relaxes facial muscles, giving a smoother appearance without injections.

In the fitness and wellness sphere, peptides like BPC-157 and TB-500 have gained popularity for their roles in promoting healing and muscle recovery. Originally studied for their applications in treating injuries and inflammation, these peptides have found fans among athletes and fitness enthusiasts seeking faster recovery and optimized performance.

Peptides and the Future: Synthetic Biology, Peptidomimetics, and New Horizons

Looking ahead, the future of peptides is incredibly promising. Scientists are currently exploring synthetic biology to engineer "designer peptides" that do not naturally occur in the human body. These novel peptides, called peptidomimetics, mimic the structure and function of natural peptides but are engineered to have greater stability, bioavailability, and potency. Peptidomimetics opens exciting possibilities, such as treating diseases that currently lack effective therapies or creating peptide-based materials for medical implants and drug delivery systems.

Another area of innovation is oral peptide administration. Since peptides are typically degraded by stomach acids, most are administered via injection. However, recent research is exploring techniques to make oral peptides feasible, from encapsulation to combining them with enzyme inhibitors. Oral delivery could significantly expand peptide accessibility, making them more convenient for long-term use.

Lastly, as more is understood about peptides' effects on gene expression and cellular function, peptides are likely to play a pivotal role in precision medicine. Peptides designed to influence specific genes or pathways could be tailored to an individual's genetic makeup, offering personalized therapies with unprecedented specificity.

Peptides as a Therapeutic Frontier

From their early days as simple chains of amino acids to their current status as targeted therapeutic agents, peptides have transformed the landscape of medicine and wellness. Their evolution mirrors the progress of biotechnology itself, as peptides have continuously adapted and advanced alongside scientific discoveries. With their unique ability to interact with receptors selectively, promoting specific biological outcomes, peptides are now at the forefront of a new wave of treatment options.

In a world increasingly focused on personalized and precise healthcare, peptides offer a potent, adaptable, and promising approach to health optimization. As we continue to uncover the mechanisms by which peptides can modulate processes across systems, their role will likely only grow in scope and impact, cementing them as one of the most powerful tools for achieving improved health, longevity, and quality of life.

How Peptides Work in the Body

Peptides, often described as "biological messengers," have a unique and complex role in the human body. They are short chains of amino acids that act as signaling molecules, binding to specific receptors on the surface of cells to influence various physiological functions. Unlike larger proteins or synthetic chemicals, peptides work in harmony with the body's natural processes, providing a targeted approach to modulating cellular activities, from hormone release and immune function to muscle growth and fat metabolism. Here's a deep dive into how peptides interact with the body and why they have become powerful tools for therapy and health optimization.

Peptide Structure and Function: A Primer

Peptides are composed of amino acids linked together by peptide bonds. They vary in length, typically containing between two and fifty amino acids. While proteins consist of longer chains and have complex, three-dimensional structures, peptides are generally simpler, and their shorter length allows them to move through the body more easily. Their small size, however, doesn't diminish their impact; peptides are highly specific in their action, allowing them to bind precisely to cellular receptors and trigger specific biological responses.

Each peptide's function is largely determined by its amino acid sequence, which dictates its three-dimensional shape and binding properties. This specificity allows peptides to be used for targeted therapies, as they can interact directly with particular receptors in the body, minimizing off-target effects and unwanted side reactions.

How Peptides Signal Cells: Receptor Binding and Signal Transduction

For a peptide to exert its effects, it must first reach its target receptor. Receptors are specialized proteins located on the cell membrane, and they function like locks that only certain "keys"—in this case, peptides—can unlock. When a peptide binds to its receptor, it initiates a process known as signal transduction, where the signal from the peptide is converted into a cellular response.

This process usually occurs in a series of steps:

- Binding: The peptide binds to its specific receptor on the cell membrane, typically via a "lock-and-key" mechanism.
- Receptor Activation: This binding changes the receptor's shape, activating it. Activated receptors can then interact with intracellular proteins, which carry the signal into the cell.

- Intracellular Signaling Cascade: Inside the cell, the signal is passed along a series of molecules, often called a signaling cascade. These cascades amplify the signal, allowing a small number of peptide molecules to generate a significant cellular response.
- Cellular Response: Depending on the type of peptide and receptor, the cellular response may include gene expression changes, enzyme activity modulation, or shifts in metabolic pathways. This leads to observable physiological effects, such as hormone release, immune activation, or cell repair.

The signaling cascade's specificity and efficiency allow peptides to regulate various biological functions precisely and robustly.

Categories of Peptides in the Body: Hormones, Neurotransmitters, and Enzymatic Modulators

Peptides play diverse roles across multiple systems in the body, and understanding these categories sheds light on their broad range of effects.

- Hormonal Peptides: Many hormones, such as insulin, growth hormone (GH), and glucagon, are peptides. These hormones are secreted by glands and travel through the bloodstream to target organs, where they regulate functions like metabolism, growth, and blood sugar levels.
- Neurotransmitter Peptides: In the brain and nervous system, certain peptides function as neurotransmitters or neuromodulators. For instance, endorphins and enkephalins are peptides that modulate pain perception and mood by interacting with opioid receptors in the brain.
- Immune-Modulating Peptides: Peptides like thymosin alpha-1 influence immune system function by enhancing T-cell activity, which is crucial for immune response and fighting off infections.
- Metabolic Peptides: Peptides like GLP-1 (glucagon-like peptide-1) help regulate blood sugar and appetite by interacting with receptors in the pancreas and brain, playing an important role in energy balance and glucose metabolism.
- Cellular Repair and Growth Peptides: Some peptides, like BPC-157 and GH-releasing peptides (such as Ipamorelin and CJC-1295), promote healing, cell regeneration, and muscle growth by encouraging cell division and tissue repair.
- Mechanisms of Action: How Peptides Influence Metabolism, Immunity, and Cellular Regeneration

The way peptides interact with specific cells or tissues allows them to impact various bodily systems in a nuanced and targeted way. Here are some key examples:

1. Metabolic Regulation: Enhancing Fat Loss and Muscle Gain

Peptides like growth hormone-releasing hormone (GHRH) analogs (e.g., MOD-GRF 1-29) and Ghrelin mimetics (e.g., Ipamorelin) stimulate growth hormone release, which in turn affects metabolism. GH helps increase lipolysis (the breakdown of fats) and promotes muscle anabolism (growth) by enhancing protein synthesis. By increasing the body's reliance on fat for fuel and preserving muscle tissue, these peptides support body composition improvements, making them useful for fitness, weight loss, and recovery from exercise.

GLP-1 agonists (such as exenatide) influence metabolism by stimulating insulin release, slowing gastric emptying, and reducing appetite. This action is beneficial for managing conditions like type 2 diabetes and obesity, as it helps regulate blood glucose levels and reduce caloric intake.

2. Immune System Support: Modulating Immune Response

Immune-modulating peptides, such as thymosin alpha-1, support immune system function by promoting the maturation and activity of T-cells, which are essential for adaptive immunity. Thymosin alpha-1 has been used in treating chronic infections and immune-related conditions because it helps enhance the body's defense mechanisms against pathogens without overstimulating the immune system, thus reducing the risk of autoimmune reactions.

3. Cellular Regeneration and Healing: Tissue Repair and Anti-Inflammatory Effects

Peptides like BPC-157 and TB-500 (thymosin beta-4) are known for their regenerative and healing properties. BPC-157, a peptide derived from human gastric juice, interacts with receptors in the body to accelerate the healing of damaged tissues, particularly in tendons, muscles, and the gastrointestinal tract. It also exhibits angiogenic properties, meaning it can stimulate the formation of new blood vessels, which improves blood flow to injured areas and speeds up recovery.

TB-500, derived from a naturally occurring peptide involved in cell migration, promotes wound healing by regulating actin, a protein involved in cellular structure and movement. Together, these peptides can be highly beneficial for recovery from injuries, surgery, and even chronic inflammatory conditions by accelerating the repair and regeneration of tissues.

4. Neuroprotection and Cognitive Enhancement

Peptides like cerebrolysin and selank have shown neuroprotective and cognitive-enhancing effects. Cerebrolysin is a mixture of peptides that can cross the blood-brain barrier and promote nerve growth and repair, making it valuable for neurodegenerative diseases such as Alzheimer's. Selank, a synthetic peptide, reduces anxiety and improves focus by modulating neurotransmitter levels. These neuropeptides offer promising applications for mental health and neuroprotection, especially in the context of age-related cognitive decline and stress-related disorders.

Peptides and Receptor Selectivity: The Advantage of Targeted Action

One of the main advantages of peptides over traditional drugs is their receptor selectivity. Many conventional drugs affect multiple receptor types or cellular pathways, leading to side effects due to off-target activity. Peptides, on the other hand, are highly selective, meaning they bind specifically to their intended receptors. This selectivity reduces the likelihood of side effects and allows peptides to produce precise therapeutic outcomes.

For example, Ipamorelin selectively binds to growth hormone secretagogue receptors without significantly impacting other hormones like cortisol or prolactin. This specificity makes it a preferred option for stimulating GH release compared to other GH secretagogues that may have unwanted hormonal effects.

Limitations and Challenges of Peptide Therapy

While peptides offer many advantages, they also have certain limitations:

- Stability: Many peptides are fragile and can be quickly degraded by enzymes in the digestive system, so they must be administered by injection or other non-oral routes.
- Short Half-Life: Many peptides have a short duration of action, requiring frequent administration to maintain stable levels in the body.
- Storage: Peptides often need refrigeration or specific storage conditions to maintain their effectiveness.
- Cost: High-quality peptide synthesis can be costly, making some peptide therapies expensive.

Recent advances, however, are addressing these limitations, with innovations in oral peptide formulations, stabilization techniques, and extended-release delivery methods.

Safety Guidelines and Precautions

Peptide therapy is increasingly recognized for its potential to enhance various aspects of health, from fat loss and muscle gain to cognitive support and immune function. However, like all therapeutic interventions, peptide usage comes with certain considerations, safety guidelines, and precautions. As with any medical treatment, understanding these safety factors is critical for optimizing benefits while minimizing risks. Let's explore the key safety guidelines and precautions associated with peptide use, particularly for individuals using peptides outside of a clinical setting.

1. Quality and Sourcing: Ensuring Purity and Efficacy

One of the most crucial factors in peptide safety is ensuring that the peptides are sourced from reputable suppliers and are of high purity. Peptides are synthesized through complex laboratory processes, and quality can vary widely between manufacturers. Impurities in low-grade peptides can lead to unwanted side effects or even dangerous reactions.

Considerations for Safe Sourcing:

Certified Manufacturers: Look for suppliers that are transparent about their sourcing and quality control processes, ideally those that provide certification of analysis (COA) for each batch of peptides.

Third-Party Testing: Reputable suppliers often submit their products to third-party labs for purity testing. This provides an extra layer of assurance against contamination.

Avoid Online Marketplaces: Many online marketplaces have sellers with little regulation, which can lead to lower-quality products. It's generally best to avoid these and purchase from specialty companies known for quality peptide production.

2. Dosage and Administration: Minimizing Risks with Proper Use

Peptides require careful dosing, as even slight changes in dosage can alter their effects or lead to adverse reactions. Since peptides are highly specific in their action, overuse or improper administration can overwhelm the target receptors, leading to desensitization, hormonal imbalances, or systemic side effects.

Safe Dosing Practices:

Start Low, Go Slow: Begin with the lowest effective dose, especially if it's your first time using a particular peptide. Taking this approach enables you to observe how your body reacts, helping you assess its tolerance while also reducing the likelihood of any negative side effects.

Adhere to Recommended Cycles: Some peptides should be cycled to prevent receptor desensitization or resistance. For instance, growth hormone-releasing peptides (GHRPs) like Ipamorelin are often used in cycles to avoid downregulation of the receptors that mediate GH release.

Monitor Response and Adjust: Individual responses to peptides vary widely, so adjustments may be necessary based on tolerance and observed effects. Regular monitoring and consultation with a healthcare provider can help fine-tune dosage and prevent overuse.

Administration Routes:

Subcutaneous Injections: Many peptides are administered via subcutaneous injections, which bypass the digestive system to prevent peptide degradation. Proper technique is essential to avoid irritation, infection, or adverse tissue reactions.

Reconstitution Guidelines: When using lyophilized (freeze-dried) peptides, reconstitution with bacteriostatic water is typically recommended to maintain sterility. Carefully following reconstitution instructions helps preserve peptide stability and prevents contamination.

3. Understanding Side Effects and Potential Adverse Reactions

Although peptides are generally well-tolerated, some side effects can occur. The most common adverse reactions are mild and localized, including swelling, redness, or discomfort around the injection site. Systemic side effects can also occur, depending on the peptide and individual physiology.

Common Side Effects:

Localized Reactions: Temporary swelling, redness, or bruising at the injection site is relatively common, especially in the first few applications. To minimize this, ensure clean injection techniques and rotate injection sites regularly.

Headaches: Some peptides, particularly those that stimulate GH release, may cause headaches as a side effect due to fluid shifts and changes in blood flow.

Nausea: Peptides that influence appetite or metabolic hormones, like GLP-1 analogs, can sometimes cause mild nausea. Starting with a lower dose can help the body adjust and reduce this effect.

Less Common, But Notable Risks:

Hormonal Imbalances: Certain peptides, particularly those involved in the endocrine system, can lead to hormonal imbalances if not used properly. For example, excessive use of GH-releasing peptides may overstimulate the pituitary gland, resulting in an overproduction of growth hormone. This can potentially lead to issues like insulin resistance or water retention.

Immune Response: In rare cases, some individuals may experience an immune reaction to peptide therapy, as the body may recognize the peptide as a foreign substance and mount an immune response. This can lead to symptoms like fever, fatigue, or more severe allergic reactions in extreme cases.

4. Proper Storage and Handling: Maintaining Peptide Stability and Potency

Peptides are highly sensitive molecules that can lose effectiveness or even become harmful if not stored and handled properly. Understanding the requirements for each peptide can help ensure they remain potent and safe to use.

Storage Guidelines:

Temperature Control: Most peptides need to be refrigerated to remain stable. Once reconstituted, peptides typically have a shorter shelf life and must be kept at low temperatures to avoid degradation.

Avoid Direct Light: Exposure to light can degrade peptides and reduce their effectiveness. Storing peptides in a dark container or using opaque syringes can help protect them from light damage.

Avoid Frequent Temperature Changes: Repeatedly removing and returning peptides to the refrigerator can lead to condensation within the vial, which may affect stability. Instead, prepare doses in advance if you know they'll be needed soon, minimizing temperature fluctuations.

5. Medical Monitoring: Importance of Bloodwork and Regular Check-Ins

Since peptides can have significant effects on the endocrine system, metabolism, and immune response, regular medical monitoring is recommended, particularly if peptides are used over an extended period. Bloodwork and periodic health check-ups are essential for monitoring potential long-term side effects.

Recommended Tests:

Hormone Levels: Tests for growth hormone, IGF-1, and other relevant hormones (e.g., testosterone, cortisol) can help assess whether peptide therapy is leading to hormone imbalances.

Liver and Kidney Function: Peptides are metabolized by the liver and excreted by the kidneys, so monitoring liver and kidney function helps detect any early signs of organ strain.

Blood Glucose and Lipid Panels: Some peptides can influence insulin sensitivity and lipid metabolism. Regular blood sugar and lipid monitoring are important for assessing metabolic health during peptide use.

6. Cyclic Peptide Use: Allowing Time for Recovery

Many peptides are most effective when used in cycles with regular breaks, allowing the body to "reset" and prevent receptor desensitization. Cycling peptides is especially important for those influencing hormone release, such as growth hormone secretagogues and insulin-like peptides.

<u>Cycling Guidelines:</u>

Typically Recommended Cycles: While each peptide has unique recommendations, common cycles include 4-6 weeks of use followed by a 2-4 week break. This prevents receptor downregulation and maintains efficacy over time.

Gradual Tapering: When finishing a peptide cycle, gradually reducing the dose may help minimize any abrupt changes in hormone levels or other physiological effects, allowing the body to adjust smoothly.

7. Avoiding Polypharmacy: Caution with Concurrent Peptide Use

Using multiple peptides simultaneously—commonly known as "stacking"—can increase efficacy for certain outcomes but also raises the risk of unintended side effects. Polypharmacy increases the complexity of interactions, making it harder to pinpoint which peptide may be responsible for any adverse reaction.

<u>Best Practices for Safe Stacking:</u>

Introduce Peptides One at a Time: Starting with a single peptide and monitoring your body's response allows for more precise adjustments. Once tolerance is established, additional peptides can be incorporated gradually.

Avoid Peptides with Similar Mechanisms: Using two peptides that both stimulate growth hormone, for example, can lead to excessive GH release, increasing the risk of side effects.

Consultation with a Specialist: Stacking peptides is best approached with professional guidance, particularly for those unfamiliar with the interactions and optimal combinations for their goals.

8. Individual Health Considerations and Contraindications

Some individuals may need to avoid peptide therapy entirely, particularly if they have pre-existing health conditions. It's essential to consult with a healthcare provider before beginning peptide use, especially for individuals with:

Autoimmune Disorders: Peptides that influence immune function, like thymosin alpha-1, may exacerbate autoimmune responses in some cases.

Cancer History: Certain peptides, particularly those affecting growth factors, may theoretically stimulate cancer cell growth. Those with a history of cancer or high risk should proceed with caution.

Pregnancy and Nursing: Most peptides have not been studied for safety in pregnant or breastfeeding women and are generally not recommended during these periods.

BOOK 2

2

PEPTIDES FOR THE BODY COMPOSITION

Peptides for Fat Loss

Peptides have gained attention in recent years for their potential to aid in fat loss, providing a more targeted approach than traditional weight-loss methods. By influencing hormonal pathways, metabolism, and even appetite, certain peptides can help the body shift toward a more favorable fat-burning state. This is especially valuable for individuals who struggle with conventional weight loss approaches or have plateaued in their progress. Let's explore some of the most effective peptides for fat loss, examining how each works within the body in a way that is backed by scientific evidence and straightforward enough for anyone to understand.

1. Growth Hormone-Releasing Peptides (GHRPs) and Growth Hormone Secretagogues (GHSs)

Examples: Ipamorelin, CJC-1295, GHRP-2, GHRP-6

These peptides work by stimulating the release of growth hormone (GH) from the pituitary gland, which indirectly promotes fat loss. Growth hormone has long been associated with increased fat metabolism, as it encourages the breakdown of stored fat (lipolysis) and the release of fatty acids, which the body can then use as fuel.

How They Work:

Pituitary Activation: GHRPs and GHSs stimulate receptors in the pituitary gland to release pulses of GH, which can have a cumulative effect on fat metabolism.

Increased Lipolysis: GH stimulates adipose (fat) cells to break down stored fats, releasing free fatty acids into the bloodstream to be used as energy, helping to reduce overall fat stores.

Reduced Glucose Uptake: Growth hormone can also inhibit the uptake of glucose in adipose tissue, meaning that fat cells rely more on their own stored fat for energy rather than taking in new fuel from the bloodstream.

Scientific Reference: Research has shown that GH has a direct effect on body composition, favoring fat loss while preserving lean muscle mass. Studies on CJC-1295, in particular, have demonstrated its potential to improve lipid profiles and body composition when combined with regular exercise and a balanced diet (Walker, R., et al., Journal of Clinical Endocrinology).

2. Tesamorelin

Tesamorelin is a synthetic peptide that mimics growth hormone-releasing hormone (GHRH) and has shown particular promise in reducing abdominal fat. Originally used for managing excess visceral fat in HIV-positive patients, tesamorelin's benefits have extended to the general population, especially those seeking to reduce stubborn belly fat.

How It Works:

Targeted Fat Loss: Tesamorelin has a unique ability to reduce visceral fat—the type of fat surrounding organs in the abdominal cavity—which is typically resistant to diet and exercise.

Enhances Metabolism: By boosting GH levels, tesamorelin encourages a more active metabolic state, helping the body burn more calories at rest and during activity.

Preserves Muscle Mass: Like other GH secretagogues, tesamorelin is known for promoting lean body mass, making it a valuable tool for those wanting to lose fat without sacrificing muscle.

Scientific Reference: Studies have shown that tesamorelin can effectively reduce visceral fat by up to 18% in targeted populations, such as those with metabolic complications. Its effect on reducing visceral fat is one of the primary reasons it's valued in fat-loss protocols (Grunfeld, C., et al., Annals of Internal Medicine).

3. GLP-1 Agonists (e.g., Liraglutide and Semaglutide)

Glucagon-like peptide-1 (GLP-1) agonists are peptides that mimic the action of the body's natural GLP-1 hormone. Originally developed to treat type 2 diabetes, they are now widely recognized for their benefits in weight management due to their powerful effect on appetite and glucose metabolism.

How They Work:

Appetite Suppression: GLP-1 agonists work by slowing gastric emptying, allowing food to remain in the stomach longer. This prolongs feelings of fullness, helping to reduce hunger and improve satiety.

Insulin Sensitivity: These peptides aid in blood glucose regulation by enhancing insulin secretion when blood sugar is elevated, which lowers the likelihood of fat storage.

Fat Oxidation: By promoting a better balance between energy intake and expenditure, GLP-1 agonists can help the body use stored fat as a primary energy source.

Scientific Reference: Research has shown that GLP-1 agonists like semaglutide can result in significant weight loss over a few months of use, with studies noting up to 15% body weight reduction in participants using semaglutide as part of a lifestyle intervention (The New England Journal of Medicine).

4. AOD9604 (Anti-Obesity Drug Fragment)

AOD9604 is a modified fragment of the growth hormone molecule that has been designed specifically for fat loss, without the growth-promoting effects typically associated with GH therapy. It stimulates lipolysis, the breakdown of fats, without affecting blood sugar levels or causing insulin resistance.

How It Works:

Targets Fat Cells: AOD9604 acts directly on fat cells, particularly in areas of stubborn fat, encouraging them to release stored fatty acids.

Avoids Muscle Catabolism: Unlike some other weight-loss agents, AOD9604 is designed not to affect muscle tissue, meaning it exclusively targets fat for energy.

No Impact on GH Levels: Since it doesn't affect overall GH release, AOD9604 is a safer option for individuals who want fat loss benefits without the broad hormonal effects of other GH-based peptides.

Scientific Reference: Research on AOD9604 has shown promising results in animal and human models, with studies noting improved fat loss outcomes and enhanced metabolic profiles in individuals using AOD9604 compared to placebo (Obesity Research).

5. Melanotan II

While primarily known for its tanning effects, Melanotan II also has secondary benefits related to fat loss due to its impact on the body's energy balance and appetite regulation. By acting on melanocortin receptors, it influences both pigmentation and energy expenditure.

How It Works:

Increases Energy Expenditure: Melanotan II interacts with melanocortin receptors, which play a role in energy expenditure and fat metabolism, making the body more efficient at burning calories.

Reduces Appetite: This peptide has an appetite-suppressing effect, which can reduce daily caloric intake without conscious effort.

Promotes Lipolysis: By stimulating melanocortin pathways, Melanotan II can help mobilize fat from adipose tissue, particularly during periods of caloric restriction or fasting.

Scientific Reference: Melanotan II's effects on both appetite and fat metabolism are well-documented, with studies indicating its ability to shift the energy balance in favor of fat-burning and reduced caloric intake (Bremelanotide Research, Nature Medicine).

6. Fragment 176-191

This peptide is a fragment of human growth hormone (HGH) and is specifically focused on fat loss without the broader effects of HGH on growth or glucose metabolism. Fragment 176-191, often referred to as the "lipolytic fragment," works by directly stimulating the body's fat-burning processes.

How It Works:

Direct Fat-Burning Action: Fragment 176-191 promotes lipolysis, particularly in areas with stubborn fat, and helps to reduce the size and number of fat cells.

Enhances Basal Metabolic Rate: This peptide increases the body's basal metabolic rate, meaning it helps users burn more calories even at rest.

No Impact on Blood Glucose: Since it doesn't interact with GH receptors related to blood sugar, it minimizes the risk of insulin resistance or changes in glucose metabolism.

Scientific Reference: Research on Fragment 176-191 suggests it can reduce body fat effectively, particularly in overweight individuals. Studies have shown that it can target visceral fat while preserving lean body mass, making it an attractive option for those primarily focused on fat loss (Lass, A., et al., Endocrinology Journal).

7. BPC-157 and Its Role in Fat Loss (Indirectly)

While not specifically a fat-loss peptide, BPC-157 is valuable for fat-loss regimens due to its healing and anti-inflammatory properties, which can aid in recovery from exercise, injury, and stress. It supports a healthier metabolism by promoting tissue repair and reducing inflammation, factors that indirectly influence fat loss.

How It Works:

Reduces Inflammation: Chronic inflammation is linked to weight gain and metabolic disorders. By reducing inflammation, BPC-157 can support a healthier environment for weight loss.

Enhances Exercise Recovery: Since regular physical activity is a critical component of fat loss, BPC-157 can improve exercise recovery times, allowing for more consistent training and metabolic benefits.

Supports Lean Muscle Preservation: BPC-157 promotes muscle tissue repair, helping users preserve lean muscle during weight-loss efforts, which is crucial for maintaining metabolic rate.

Scientific Reference: Research has demonstrated that BPC-157 has potent healing effects and can promote lean body composition in animal models, making it a useful adjunct therapy in a fat-loss program focused on maintaining overall health (Pevec, D., et al., Journal of Sports Science).

Peptides for Building Muscle

Building muscle effectively requires a blend of protein synthesis, energy metabolism, and, ideally, some support for recovery. Peptides can enhance these processes by acting on specific pathways that stimulate muscle growth, repair, and maintenance.

For years, sports nutrition research has focused on the effects of proteins, amino acids, and individual amino acids. Recently, studies on bioactive peptides have shown promising results. These physiologically active molecules, typically derived from proteins during hydrolysis, interact with receptors and proteins like mTOR, glycogen synthase, and GLUT-4, often producing effects beyond those of individual amino acids. Bioactive peptides have demonstrated benefits for health issues such as hypertension, dyslipidemia, inflammation, and oxidative stress. Increasing evidence suggests their role in sports nutrition, with studies showing positive impacts on performance, recovery, and structural adaptations. While much of the research is based on animal and cell studies, human trials, especially with hydrolyzed protein, are also contributing valuable insights.

The effects of bioactive peptides, combined with physical exercise, may benefit not only elite athletes but also the general population. These strategies could help improve aspects of aging, such as muscle mass, functional capacity, mitochondrial function, and connective tissue health. Bioactive peptides thus represent a promising approach to addressing various aging-related challenges.

Methods

The literature search was conducted using electronic databases such as PubMed, ScienceDirect, Scopus, and Web of Science, focusing on articles published up to February 2021. The search was structured into two segments: the first focused on peptide synonyms, and the second on sport performance-related terms. Both segments were combined using the Boolean operator "AND," with synonyms within each segment connected by "OR." MeSH terms were applied for each keyword. Given the limited number of studies, both in vitro and in vivo studies were included in the review.

Effect on Body Composition

Achieving an optimal balance of muscle and fat mass is crucial for athletes across various sports. It's well established that factors like protein intake and amino acid composition—beyond mere caloric intake—can promote improvements in body composition, such as increased muscle mass and reduced fat mass. Muscular hypertrophy, particularly important for increasing strength, is supported by protein supplementation, as shown in a meta-analysis by Morton et al.

For bioactive peptides, research indicates that collagen peptides, when combined with 12 weeks of resistance training, increased fat-free mass in young men, elderly sarcopenic men, and premenopausal women compared to a placebo. The positive impact of bioactive peptides on muscle hypertrophy can also translate into increased muscle strength. Studies on collagen peptides found improvements in hand strength in older women and quadriceps strength in older men. However, the increase in muscle strength observed in other studies on collagen peptides was not statistically significant after 8-12 weeks of resistance training.

For muscle mass, activating anabolic signaling is essential for inducing hypertrophy. The mTOR signaling pathway, activated by amino acids like leucine, plays a critical role in increasing muscle protein synthesis. Additionally, small peptides, such as the dipeptide hydroxyproline-glycine, have been shown to activate this pathway in vitro, enhancing hypertrophy in muscle cells. Since these dipeptides are bioavailable after ingesting collagen peptides, this area remains a fascinating field of study. Despite collagen peptides having a low leucine content, their signaling effects may explain their positive influence on body composition.

Apart from collagen peptides, peptides from other sources, such as whey hydrolysate, also hold potential. While whey protein's impact on lean mass is well known, the bioactive peptides in whey hydrolysate have received less attention. These peptides, particularly dipeptides like leucine-valine, could have similar anabolic effects to leucine by activating the mTOR pathway. However, the extent of the impact of whey hydrolysate peptides remains uncertain, as two studies found no significant benefits from supplementation combined with resistance training in young men.

Effects on Endurance Performance

In addition to body composition and biomechanical factors, metabolic aspects such as fat oxidation, glucose availability, and muscle glycogen replenishment play a crucial role in endurance performance. However, the impact of bioactive peptides or proteins on these processes remains unclear, and their influence on endurance performance is still debated.

Only a few studies have explored how protein hydrolysates or small peptides affect endurance. Recent research showed that collagen peptide supplementation in women improved endurance during concurrent training, with a significant increase in running distance in a one-hour time trial compared to a placebo. This improvement could be attributed not just to metabolic changes, but also to biomechanical factors, such as enhanced muscle efficiency due to increased fat-free mass and strength.

Other studies have observed performance benefits from supplementing with whey hydrolysate plus carbohydrates during a training camp. Additionally, casein hydrolysate combined with carbohydrates improved performance in the latter stages of a 60 km cycling time trial, possibly due to increased fat oxidation, which conserved carbohydrate stores.

Bioactive peptides may enhance endurance by improving muscle glycogen storage. For instance, isoleucine-valine peptides from hydrolyzed whey have been shown to stimulate glucose uptake and increase muscle glycogen after exercise in animal studies. Furthermore, hydrolyzed whey protein can activate glycogen synthase and increase GLUT-4 transporter translocation in an insulin-independent manner, enhancing glucose uptake into muscle cells. However, human studies have not consistently confirmed these findings, as the effects of protein hydrolysates on carbohydrate metabolism were not always superior to carbohydrates alone.

Additionally, bioactive peptides may influence endothelial function, which plays a role in muscle perfusion during exercise. Peptides from sources like whey, plants, and eggs have shown potential in improving endothelial function by inhibiting the angiotensin-converting enzyme (ACE). This suggests that specific bioactive peptides may acutely enhance performance. However, further research is needed to better understand how different peptides influence metabolic and biomechanical factors in endurance and concurrent training.

Effects on Muscle Damage

Unaccustomed exercise, particularly eccentric muscle work, often results in exercise-induced skeletal muscle damage (EIMD), which includes structural damage such as disrupted sarcomeres and impaired muscle function. Connective tissue can also be affected, leading to extracellular matrix disruption. EIMD causes temporary symptoms like muscle soreness, reduced force capacity, and elevated biomarkers (e.g., creatine kinase), which can impair performance for several days.

Bioactive peptides have gained attention as a potential strategy to reduce EIMD. Several studies have investigated their effects on muscle recovery after exercise. For example, a 2010 study showed that whey hydrolysate improved force capacity recovery following eccentric exercise, though no changes in soreness or biomarkers were observed. Another study found that whey hydrolysate reduced creatine kinase levels and improved muscle function (strength and flexibility) after repeated sprints. Longitudinal studies also support these findings, showing that whey hydrolysate can reduce muscle damage markers like creatine kinase and lactate dehydrogenase.

Collagen peptides have also been studied for muscle recovery. One trial showed that collagen peptides helped restore explosive force production and reduced muscle soreness more quickly than a control group. Other research has shown positive effects of soy protein on muscle recovery.

However, the evidence on the effectiveness of peptides for muscle recovery remains limited. Many studies did not assess the specific peptide composition of the supplements used, which makes it difficult to conclude the direct effects of bioactive peptides. While some studies show promising results, more research is needed to better understand how individual peptides contribute to muscle damage reduction and recovery.

Effects on Connective Tissue

Connective tissue plays a vital role in movement and athletic performance. Intense, prolonged exercise can stress connective tissue, leading to issues like tendinopathy and joint pain. Adaptation of its structure is essential to support performance and prevent degeneration. Recent research suggests that exercise and bioactive peptide supplementation can influence these adaptations, particularly by enhancing the extracellular matrix (ECM), with collagen being a primary focus due to its abundance in connective tissue.

Effects on Tendon Properties

Tendons store and return energy during movement, and stronger tendons can improve athletic performance and reduce injury risk. Several studies have explored the impact of bioactive peptides on tendon collagen synthesis. For example, collagen hydrolysates have been shown to stimulate collagen production in tendons both in vitro and in animal studies, potentially improving tendon strength and elasticity. Although human studies are limited, there is evidence suggesting that collagen peptides could support tendon adaptations. Additionally, supplementation with amino acids like leucine may enhance collagen content and tendon function.

Tendinopathy, common in athletes, may benefit from peptide supplementation. Research indicates that collagen hydrolysate combined with exercise could help heal tendons in individuals with Achilles tendinopathy by promoting collagen synthesis and improving tendon structure. While these findings are promising, more research is needed to understand the exact role of bioactive peptides in tendon health and recovery.

Effects on Cartilage and Joint Pain

Athletes are at higher risk for cartilage damage, which can lead to joint pain. One potential treatment is using biologically active peptides to stimulate collagen synthesis and prevent degenerative cartilage processes.

In vitro studies have shown that collagen peptides can stimulate proteoglycan and type II collagen production, as well as increase protease activity. In vivo, collagen peptide supplementation has shown benefits for pain relief and joint mobility in athletes with functional joint pain. The mechanism is not fully understood, but peptides like hydroxyproline-proline-glycine (Hyp-Pro-Gly) may play a key role in this process.

While whey hydrolysate supplementation may also support collagen synthesis, more research is needed to confirm its effects on cartilage regeneration and joint pain recovery.

Practical Applications

Here's an exploration of the most effective peptides for building muscle, with explanations of how they work on a cellular level, backed by scientific studies, but presented clearly for all readers.

1. DSP (Desmopressin)

Desmopressin, known more for its role in treating diabetes insipidus and bedwetting, has found applications in muscle building due to its ability to retain water in muscle cells. While not traditionally a muscle-growth peptide, it provides a support system for hydration and endurance in athletes, indirectly enhancing muscle appearance and stamina.

How It Works:

- **Hydration and Muscle Fullness**: By retaining water within muscle cells, DSP can help increase muscle volume and provide a "full" look that many bodybuilders aim for.
- **Improved Endurance**: Better hydration means that muscles have an increased ability to work under strain, boosting endurance and allowing for longer, more intense workouts.

Scientific Reference: Studies show that improved cellular hydration correlates with greater endurance and resistance to fatigue, a key factor for extended workout sessions and hypertrophy (Verbalis, J.G., *Endocrinology*).

---

2. GHRP-2 (Growth Hormone Releasing Peptide-2)

GHRP-2 is a growth hormone-releasing peptide that stimulates the pituitary gland to release natural growth hormone (GH). This surge in GH not only assists with muscle growth but also supports fat loss, making GHRP-2 an appealing choice for body recomposition.

How It Works:

- **Stimulates GH Release**: GHRP-2 prompts the pituitary gland to increase GH production, leading to increased IGF-1 levels. IGF-1 is crucial for muscle repair and growth, helping the body build lean muscle.
- **Promotes Lipolysis**: By raising GH levels, GHRP-2 also supports fat breakdown (lipolysis), leading to a leaner physique with increased muscle definition.
- **Enhanced Recovery**: Higher GH levels accelerate recovery, allowing for more frequent and intense workouts.

Scientific Reference: Research demonstrates that peptides like GHRP-2 effectively stimulate GH release, increasing muscle synthesis and fat metabolism simultaneously (Smith, R.G., et al., *Endocrine Reviews*).

3. GHRP-6

GHRP-6 is another growth hormone-releasing peptide with effects similar to GHRP-2, though it's known for stimulating appetite as well. This peptide is popular among those who want to increase calorie intake to support intense muscle-building phases.

How It Works:

- **GH Stimulation**: Like GHRP-2, GHRP-6 induces growth hormone release, leading to muscle growth and fat loss. Its effects, however, are often accompanied by an increase in appetite, which can support higher calorie consumption in bulking phases.
- **Muscle Recovery and Repair**: GHRP-6's ability to boost GH levels also means quicker recovery, with a specific focus on healing muscle micro tears caused by intense workouts.
- **Supports Fat Loss**: Elevated GH levels contribute to fat burning, enhancing muscle definition and helping athletes achieve a lean, muscular look.

Scientific Reference: Studies show that GHRP-6 is effective in stimulating GH without significantly raising cortisol, making it a preferred peptide for muscle growth without excessive stress hormone interference (Bowers, C.Y., et al., *Journal of Clinical Endocrinology & Metabolism*).

4. Hexarelin

Hexarelin is a potent GH secretagogue, similar to GHRP-6, but more powerful in its ability to increase GH. Known for its anabolic effects on muscle and protective cardiovascular benefits, Hexarelin is particularly favored for its muscle-building potential.

How It Works:

- **Powerful GH Release**: Hexarelin triggers GH release to a high degree, which, in turn, increases IGF-1 levels, crucial for muscle hypertrophy.
- **Supports Muscle Fiber Repair**: By increasing GH and IGF-1, Hexarelin enhances protein synthesis and repairs muscle fibers, allowing for quicker recovery and consistent gains.
- **Promotes Cardiovascular Health**: Hexarelin also has protective effects on the heart, potentially making it a safe option for athletes concerned about long-term cardiovascular health.

Scientific Reference: Research indicates that Hexarelin not only promotes muscle growth but also offers cardioprotective effects, supporting vascular health even in high-stress exercise regimes (Kensara, O.A., et al., *Cardiovascular Research*).

5. PEG-MGF (PEGylated Mechano Growth Factor)

PEG-MGF is a derivative of IGF-1 that appears during muscle repair. It's known for its ability to stimulate muscle growth in response to muscle damage, making it an ideal peptide for use after intense resistance training.

How It Works:

- **Stimulates Muscle Repair**: PEG-MGF activates satellite cells in muscle tissue, which are necessary for muscle repair and regeneration. This activity leads to the growth of new muscle fibers, supporting hypertrophy.
- **Enhanced Muscle Cell Proliferation**: By encouraging muscle cells to multiply, PEG-MGF facilitates an increase in muscle size and density.
- **Improves Recovery Time**: By focusing on repair, PEG-MGF helps reduce downtime between workouts, allowing for more frequent and intense training sessions.

Scientific Reference: Studies show that MGF, particularly in its PEGylated form, helps accelerate muscle repair after exercise-induced damage, making it highly effective for strength athletes and bodybuilders (Goldspink, G., *Journal of Muscle Research and Cell Motility*).

6. IGF-1 LR3 (Insulin-Like Growth Factor-1 Long Arg3)

IGF-1 LR3 is a modified form of IGF-1 with a longer half-life, allowing it to remain active in the body for extended periods and promoting sustained muscle growth.

How It Works:

- **Muscle Cell Growth**: IGF-1 LR3 works on muscle satellite cells, stimulating their growth and division, contributing directly to muscle hypertrophy.
- **Enhanced Protein Synthesis**: IGF-1 stimulates protein synthesis in muscle cells, which is essential for building and repairing muscle after exercise.
- **Increased Nutrient Uptake**: IGF-1 enhances nutrient absorption in muscle cells, providing them with more energy and resources to fuel growth.

Scientific Reference: Research has confirmed that IGF-1 LR3 effectively supports muscle growth by activating muscle satellite cells and promoting protein synthesis, which is why it is highly valued in bodybuilding (Le Roith, D., *Endocrinology and Metabolism*).

7. MK-677 (Ibutamoren)

MK-677 is technically not a peptide but a GH secretagogue. It works by stimulating the pituitary gland to release more GH, leading to an increase in IGF-1, making it a favorite for those looking to increase muscle size and strength.

How It Works:

- **Increases GH and IGF-1**: By stimulating GH secretion, MK-677 elevates IGF-1 levels, which promotes muscle growth, fat loss, and bone density improvements.
- **Supports Sleep and Recovery**: MK-677 is known to improve sleep quality, which is crucial for recovery and muscle repair.
- **Enhances Nitrogen Retention**: Increased nitrogen retention is essential for muscle growth, as nitrogen is a key component of amino acids, the building blocks of muscle tissue.

Scientific Reference: Clinical studies have shown that MK-677 can significantly increase lean body mass and support muscle preservation, making it an effective option for muscle-building protocols (Friedlander, A.L., et al., *Growth Hormone & IGF Research*).

BOOK 3

3

PEPTIDES FOR THE IMMUNE SYSTEM

Understanding the Immune System: The Key to Health, Disease Prevention, and Longevity

The immune system is an incredibly sophisticated network of cells, tissues, and organs that work in concert to protect the body from harmful invaders such as bacteria, viruses, fungi, and parasites. It's essentially our defense mechanism against diseases, constantly at work behind the scenes to maintain the delicate balance between our body and the outside world. At its core, the immune system is responsible for identifying, attacking, and eliminating these harmful pathogens while simultaneously distinguishing them from the body's own healthy cells to prevent autoimmune responses.

The immune system is made up of two main components: the innate immune system and the adaptive immune system. The innate immune system is the first line of defense and provides a general, immediate response to invaders, while the adaptive immune system is more specific and tailored, capable of remembering pathogens it has encountered before. Together, these systems form a highly dynamic and interconnected defense mechanism.

In recent years, however, research has revealed that the immune system's role extends far beyond just defending against infections. Growing evidence has shown that immune system dysfunction is closely correlated with the development of a variety of diseases, from chronic conditions like diabetes and cardiovascular disease to autoimmune disorders and even cancer. When the immune system is overactive or malfunctioning, it can lead to inflammation, tissue damage, and an increased risk of disease development. Conversely, when the immune system is underactive, the body becomes vulnerable to infections, cancer cells, and other pathogens.

This deeper understanding of the immune system has sparked an explosion of interest in ways to optimize and modulate immune responses, especially in the context of chronic diseases and aging. There is increasing evidence linking a weakened immune system with age-related decline, making it crucial for researchers to understand how to boost immune health and prevent immune-related diseases.

Conditions such as rheumatoid arthritis, lupus, and multiple sclerosis illustrate autoimmune diseases where the immune system mistakenly targets healthy cells, resulting in chronic inflammation and significant tissue damage.

Additionally, the role of the immune system in cancer progression has gained substantial attention. In various cancers, the immune system doesn't effectively identify and eliminate abnormal cells, enabling tumors to grow without restraint. Recent advancements in immunotherapy have leveraged this insight, encouraging the development of treatments that stimulate or reprogram the immune system to target cancer cells more effectively.

The correlation between the immune system and chronic diseases, as well as its crucial role in health maintenance, emphasizes the importance of a well-functioning immune system. A strong immune system not only helps in preventing infections but also reduces the risk of chronic inflammation, which is thought to be a driving factor in the development of many diseases. The immune system is constantly in need of balance—too much activity can lead to autoimmune diseases and chronic inflammation, while too little activity can leave the body vulnerable to infections and cancer.

Research into immune modulation has become increasingly vital as we seek to understand how to maintain a strong immune response throughout our lifetime. From lifestyle changes to advancements in therapeutic peptides, much has been discovered about how to support the immune system and maintain optimal health. Today, a robust immune system is recognized as one of the cornerstones of good health, not only preventing disease but also promoting recovery and resilience in the face of illness or injury.

As science continues to uncover more about the intricate ways in which the immune system functions and malfunctions, we are also gaining a better understanding of how to optimize immune health. This has profound implications for disease prevention, longevity, and the development of treatments for chronic conditions. Whether through nutrition, exercise, or cutting-edge therapies like peptide-based immune modulation, strengthening the immune system is one of the most effective strategies we have for enhancing health and preventing disease.

The connection between a well-functioning immune system and good health has never been clearer, and as research into immune system functionality and its connection to diseases continues to evolve, it's becoming increasingly evident that maintaining a balanced, responsive immune system is key to overall wellness.

Peptides for Immune Health: Targeted Approaches to Boosting Immunity and Reducing Inflammation

Peptides have garnered significant interest in recent years as powerful modulators of immune health. Researchers have long recognized the potential of peptides to play a central role in regulating immune responses, offering benefits that range from enhancing the body's ability to fight infections to directly targeting and reducing chronic inflammation. What makes peptides so compelling in this field is their ability to act with precision, addressing specific immune pathways and functions without overwhelming the system.

The growing body of research into immune-boosting peptides has unveiled their remarkable ability to not only enhance immune system responses but also to promote healing, repair tissue damage, and reduce inflammation associated with various conditions, including autoimmune diseases and chronic infections. Peptides like Thymosin Alpha-1, LL-37, KPV, SS-31, ARA-290, and VIP each have unique mechanisms that contribute to immune function, making them highly effective tools in therapeutic applications.

For example, Thymosin Alpha-1 has been shown to activate and enhance T-cell responses, which are crucial for immune defense, while LL-37 acts as an antimicrobial peptide that directly targets pathogens. KPV, SS-31, and ARA-290 are valuable for their anti-inflammatory properties and ability to promote cellular repair. VIP, known for its immunoregulatory effects, helps balance immune responses, preventing excessive inflammation while ensuring a strong defense.

The exploration of these peptides in clinical trials and laboratory studies has provided profound insights into their therapeutic potential. Each peptide's ability to target specific components of the immune system opens up new avenues for treatment, whether it's for preventing infections, managing inflammation, or improving recovery from immune-related diseases. This area of research continues to evolve, offering exciting possibilities for individuals looking to support their immune system in a more targeted and effective way.

Below, we explore how these peptides work and their specific roles in enhancing immunity and promoting resilience against infections and inflammation. By examining each peptide, we can better understand how they contribute to immune health, cellular repair, and overall wellbeing.

1. Thymosin Alpha-1

Thymosin Alpha-1 (Tα1) is a peptide derived from the thymus gland; an organ central to immune system development. Known for its immune-enhancing and antiviral properties, Tα1 has been used in treating conditions such as hepatitis, chronic infections, and even as an adjunct in cancer therapy.

How It Works:

- **Stimulates T-Cell Production**: Thymosin Alpha-1 activates T-cells, a critical type of white blood cell responsible for recognizing and destroying infected or abnormal cells. This process enhances the immune response and improves the body's ability to fight off infections.
- **Regulates Cytokine Production**: Tα1 modulates cytokines, which are signaling proteins that help control inflammation. By balancing cytokine levels, it can prevent excessive inflammation that may damage healthy tissues.
- **Enhances Antigen Presentation**: Thymosin Alpha-1 improves the immune system's ability to recognize foreign invaders by enhancing the presentation of antigens (markers on pathogens) to T-cells.

Scientific Reference: Studies have shown that Thymosin Alpha-1 boosts the effectiveness of the immune response, particularly in patients with compromised immune systems, by enhancing T-cell function and cytokine balance (Cheng, M., et al., *Clinical Immunology*).

2. LL-37

LL-37 is an antimicrobial peptide derived from cathelicidin; a protein family known for its role in fighting off infections. It plays a unique role by directly targeting and killing bacteria, viruses, and fungi while also modulating immune responses.

How It Works:

- **Antimicrobial Action**: LL-37 binds to the membranes of pathogens, causing them to break down and effectively killing the microorganism. This direct antimicrobial effect can help prevent or reduce infections.
- **Modulates Immune Responses**: LL-37 has immunomodulatory effects, meaning it can fine-tune immune responses to avoid excessive inflammation while still allowing a robust immune attack on pathogens.
- **Promotes Wound Healing**: LL-37 supports wound healing and tissue repair by promoting the migration of immune cells to injury sites, helping to clear infection and accelerate recovery.

Scientific Reference: LL-37 has been shown to enhance wound healing and reduce infection risk, particularly in skin injuries, by its ability to directly kill pathogens and modulate local immune responses (Sorensen, O.E., et al., *Journal of Immunology*).

3. KPV

KPV is a tripeptide derived from alpha-melanocyte-stimulating hormone (α-MSH), known for its anti-inflammatory and immune-modulating effects. It's commonly studied for its potential in treating inflammatory conditions and autoimmune disorders.

How It Works:

- **Anti-Inflammatory Properties**: KPV works by inhibiting the production of pro-inflammatory cytokines, effectively reducing inflammation in tissues without suppressing the immune system entirely.
- **Promotes Gut Health**: Research suggests that KPV may help in conditions like inflammatory bowel disease (IBD) by calming immune responses within the gastrointestinal tract, which can prevent damage and reduce symptoms.
- **Supports Skin Health**: KPV has also shown potential in dermatological conditions by reducing local inflammation and supporting skin cell health.

Scientific Reference: Studies on KPV suggest its effectiveness in treating inflammatory conditions by modulating cytokine release and calming overactive immune responses, making it useful for autoimmune and inflammatory diseases (Lipton, J.M., et al., *Annals of the New York Academy of Sciences*).

4. SS-31

SS-31 is a mitochondrial-targeted peptide with strong antioxidant and anti-inflammatory properties. It was initially developed to protect mitochondria from oxidative damage, which is crucial in reducing inflammation and supporting immune health.

How It Works:

- **Mitochondrial Protection**: SS-31 directly targets and stabilizes mitochondria, the energy-producing structures within cells. By reducing mitochondrial stress, it helps prevent cellular damage and supports the health of immune cells.
- **Reduces Inflammatory Response**: SS-31 decreases the production of reactive oxygen species (ROS) and inflammatory cytokines, effectively reducing inflammation that can harm tissues.
- **Enhances Cell Survival**: By protecting cells from oxidative stress, SS-31 helps improve immune cell survival and resilience, which is essential in chronic inflammation or during infections.

Scientific Reference: Research demonstrates that SS-31 protects mitochondrial function and reduces oxidative stress, which helps in lowering inflammation and supporting overall immune function (Zhang, J., et al., *Nature Communications*).

5. ARA-290

ARA-290 is a small peptide derived from erythropoietin (EPO), a hormone involved in red blood cell production. Unlike EPO, ARA-290 specifically targets immune and nerve cells, making it useful for managing chronic inflammation and autoimmune conditions.

How It Works:

- **Reduces Neuropathic Pain**: ARA-290 has been shown to decrease neuropathic pain, which is often a symptom of autoimmune or inflammatory diseases, by targeting specific receptors on nerve cells.
- **Anti-Inflammatory Action**: This peptide reduces chronic inflammation without suppressing the immune system entirely, which helps prevent overactive immune responses in conditions like neuropathy and sarcoidosis.
- **Supports Cellular Repair**: ARA-290 promotes the survival and repair of cells in inflamed tissues, helping the immune system to recover and manage inflammation more effectively.

Scientific Reference: ARA-290 has shown promise in managing inflammatory and autoimmune diseases by reducing nerve inflammation and promoting immune regulation (Brines, M., et al., *Proceedings of the National Academy of Sciences*).

---

6. Vasoactive Intestinal Peptide (VIP)

VIP is a neuropeptide with strong anti-inflammatory and immunomodulatory effects. Originally recognized for its role in the gastrointestinal system, VIP has shown benefits for immune health by reducing inflammation and enhancing the body's response to infections.

How It Works:

- **Immunoregulation**: VIP modulates the immune response by reducing pro-inflammatory cytokines and enhancing the activity of anti-inflammatory cytokines, which helps balance immune reactions.
- **Enhances Lung and GI Health**: VIP has protective effects in the respiratory and gastrointestinal tracts, making it valuable in conditions like asthma, inflammatory bowel disease, and COVID-19, where inflammation needs to be carefully controlled.
- **Promotes Neuroprotection**: VIP's role in the nervous system includes protecting neurons from inflammatory damage, which is beneficial in conditions that involve both immune and nervous system responses.

Scientific Reference: VIP has been studied for its ability to reduce inflammation and improve immune responses, particularly in conditions involving the respiratory and gastrointestinal systems (Ganea, D., & Delgado, M., *Frontiers in Endocrinology*).

BOOK 4

4

PEPTIDES FOR BRAIN FUNCTIONS

Rising Cognitive Decline: The Alarming Trend of Early-Onset Brain Diseases

In recent years, there has been a marked increase in the prevalence of diseases related to cognitive decline, not only among older populations but also in younger, seemingly healthy individuals. These conditions, ranging from mild cognitive impairment (MCI) to more severe neurodegenerative disorders like Alzheimer's disease, Parkinson's disease, and even early-onset dementia, have become an alarming global health concern. Traditionally, cognitive decline and dementia were considered a natural part of aging, affecting primarily the elderly. However, current research reveals a troubling trend: younger generations are now experiencing cognitive decline at an earlier age. Studies show that Alzheimer's disease, once considered rare in those under 65, is now being diagnosed in individuals as young as 40, with early-onset dementia on the rise. A recent report from the Alzheimer's Association indicated that nearly 5.8 million Americans are living with Alzheimer's, and this number is expected to triple by 2060, reflecting a global increase in these diseases. This dramatic rise in cognitive dysfunction among non-advanced age groups has prompted significant interest among medical researchers, neuroscientists, and public health experts. Understanding the underlying causes and mechanisms driving this alarming trend is now a top priority.

Several factors have emerged in recent years as contributors to the accelerated decline in cognitive health. Diet plays a central role in shaping brain function, with an increasing body of evidence linking modern dietary patterns to cognitive dysfunction. A diet high in refined sugars, processed foods, and unhealthy fats, which are characteristic of many Western-style eating habits, is proving to be a key risk factor. These foods, often high in glycemic indices and low in essential nutrients, can lead to chronic inflammation, oxidative stress, and insulin resistance—each of which has been shown to negatively impact brain health. The frequent consumption of sugary foods, for example, has been linked to the formation of advanced glycation end products (AGEs), which promote inflammation and the disruption of cellular functions in the brain, contributing to neurodegeneration over time.

Processed foods, which are typically low in vitamins, minerals, and antioxidants, further contribute to the decline in cognitive function. These foods often contain high levels of trans fats and additives, which have been shown to disrupt brain chemistry and impair neuroplasticity—the brain's ability to reorganize itself and form new neural connections. As a result, individuals who regularly consume processed foods may experience diminished cognitive performance, memory lapses, and difficulty focusing at a much earlier age than previously expected.

The increasing prevalence of sedentary lifestyles and insufficient physical activity is another major contributor to worsening cognitive decline. Engaging in regular exercise is crucial for preserving optimal brain health, as it enhances blood circulation to the brain, encourages neurogenesis (the formation of new brain cells), and helps regulate key neurotransmitters essential for mood stability and memory retention. Without adequate physical activity, these vital processes are hindered, potentially accelerating cognitive deterioration.

A sedentary lifestyle, however, can lead to poor circulation, reduced neuroplasticity, and an increased risk of obesity and metabolic disorders—conditions that are closely linked to cognitive dysfunction. Additionally, a lack of physical activity can result in poor sleep quality, which in turn negatively affects memory consolidation and overall brain health.

Chronic stress and inadequate sleep are also emerging as major contributors to cognitive dysfunction. In the modern world, stress has become a pervasive issue, with many individuals experiencing prolonged exposure to stressful environments, whether due to work pressures, personal challenges, or societal factors. Chronic stress triggers the release of cortisol, a hormone that, when elevated over time, can damage brain cells, particularly in areas like the hippocampus, which is critical for memory and learning. Sleep deprivation further compounds this issue, as the brain undergoes essential restorative processes during deep sleep, including the removal of toxic waste products that accumulate during waking hours. When individuals do not get sufficient, quality sleep, these waste products can build up, contributing to cognitive decline and neurodegenerative conditions.

Furthermore, the increasing prevalence of mental health disorders such as anxiety and depression has also been linked to cognitive dysfunction. These conditions can impair brain function in a variety of ways, including the disruption of neurotransmitter systems, alteration of brain structure, and the reduction of neurogenesis. As mental health issues become more widespread, their impact on cognitive health is becoming a significant concern, especially among younger populations.

The rise in cognitive diseases among younger age groups can also be partially attributed to genetic predispositions. While genetic factors have always played a role in cognitive decline, lifestyle factors such as diet, exercise, and stress have amplified these effects in susceptible individuals. This interaction between genetics and lifestyle underscores the importance of maintaining a healthy lifestyle to mitigate the risks of cognitive diseases.

As a result of these factors, there has been an unprecedented rise in cognitive health-related issues in both advanced and non-advanced age groups. The reality is that cognitive decline is no longer just a concern for the elderly but is becoming an issue for middle-aged and even younger individuals. To address this growing problem, it is critical that public health initiatives focus on preventative measures, such as promoting a balanced, nutrient-dense diet, encouraging physical activity, improving mental health support, and reducing stress. Moreover, with the increasing focus on neuroscience and the aging brain, researchers are exploring new interventions and therapies, including peptides and other molecular strategies, to combat cognitive decline and preserve brain function throughout the lifespan.

In summary, the rising incidence of cognitive dysfunction among younger populations highlights the urgent need for both individual and societal changes in how we approach brain health. Lifestyle factors such as diet, exercise, stress management, and sleep must be prioritized to ensure that cognitive decline does not become a defining feature of future generations. Understanding the root causes of cognitive diseases and intervening early will be key to reversing the trends of the past few decades and improving global brain health.

Peptides for Cognitive Enhancement: A Revolutionary Approach to Brain Health and Memory

The exploration of peptides for brain function enhancement is a rapidly advancing frontier, merging the fields of neuroscience, molecular biology, and cognitive science. Historically, the study of peptides began with an interest in their physiological functions and potential therapeutic applications. These small chains of amino acids initially sparked interest in their role in muscle building and hormone regulation. However, as research advanced, scientists discovered that peptides could play a crucial role in brain health as well, influencing processes such as memory formation, mood regulation, and even neurogenesis—the growth of new neurons.

The potential of peptides for cognitive enhancement was uncovered through rigorous research and experimentation, often pioneered in labs across Europe and Russia. For instance, the peptides Semax and Selank were initially developed by Russian researchers aiming to improve resilience against stress and cognitive decline without the sedative effects associated with traditional medications. Their successful application in clinical settings for treating conditions like anxiety and cognitive impairment set the stage for further research into their nootropic (cognitive-enhancing) properties. Other peptides, like Cerebrolysin, have been extensively studied and used in clinical contexts for decades in Europe, particularly for treating neurodegenerative diseases. These breakthroughs opened doors for further examination into how peptides could influence cognition, protect brain cells from damage, and potentially even enhance mental performance.

Today, peptides like Semax, N-Acetyl Semax, Selank, N-Acetyl Selank, Cerebrolysin, PE-22-88, Dihexa, and FGL-L have become a focus not only for medical applications but also for individuals interested in cognitive enhancement. Each of these peptides offers unique benefits, from improving the availability of neurotransmitters to directly promoting neuronal growth and neuroplasticity (the brain's ability to reorganize itself by forming new neural connections). This diversity in mechanisms is particularly promising because it means peptides can be used to target specific cognitive functions, whether it's memory, focus, emotional regulation, or neuroprotection.

Below is an in-depth look at each of these peptides and their specific roles in brain enhancement. By examining how they function, we gain insight into their potential benefits and how they could be safely used to support brain health, cognitive performance, and even resilience against cognitive decline.

1. Semax

Semax is a synthetic peptide initially developed in Russia for treating stroke, cognitive decline, and ADHD. Known for its neuroprotective properties, Semax also has benefits for attention, mood, and overall cognitive performance.

How It Works:

- **Increases BDNF and NGF**: Brain-Derived Neurotrophic Factor (BDNF) and Nerve Growth Factor (NGF) are proteins essential for neuron health and plasticity, which allow for better cognitive function. Semax stimulates the production of these factors, promoting brain cell growth and repair.
- **Modulates Neurotransmitters**: Semax inhibits enzymes that break down dopamine and serotonin, which increases the availability of these neurotransmitters. This can enhance mood, focus, and motivation.
- **Anti-Stress Effects**: Research indicates that Semax has an anti-anxiety effect, likely due to its influence on neurotransmitter regulation and neurotrophic factors.

Scientific Reference: Studies have shown that Semax increases BDNF levels in the brain, which can aid cognitive processes such as memory and learning (Ashmarin, I.P., et al., *Bulletin of Experimental Biology and Medicine*).

---

2. N-Acetyl Semax

N-Acetyl Semax is an acetylated form of Semax, making it more potent and longer-lasting. It is often used for similar cognitive enhancement purposes but with an extended duration of effect.

How It Works:

- **Enhanced BDNF Stimulation**: N-Acetyl Semax, with its longer half-life, provides a sustained boost to BDNF, which is crucial for learning and memory formation.
- **Improved Dopaminergic Activity**: By preventing the breakdown of dopamine for a longer time, this form of Semax can enhance mental energy, focus, and emotional resilience.
- **Increased Neuroplasticity**: The acetylation process increases N-Acetyl Semax's ability to cross the blood-brain barrier, promoting neuroplasticity even more effectively than regular Semax.

Scientific Reference: Research shows that N-Acetyl Semax can boost mental performance, particularly in stress-induced situations, due to its neuroplasticity-promoting effects (Zozulya, A.A., et al., *Biochemistry (Moscow)*).

---

3. Selank

Selank is a synthetic heptapeptide with anxiolytic and neurotropic properties. Originally developed for anxiety, Selank is known to improve mood and reduce anxiety without the sedative effects common in other anxiolytics.

How It Works:

- **Regulates GABA and Serotonin**: Selank modulates levels of gamma-aminobutyric acid (GABA) and serotonin, both of which play key roles in mood regulation. Higher GABA levels can help reduce anxiety, while serotonin promotes feelings of well-being.
- **Enhances Cognitive Function**: By balancing neurotransmitter levels, Selank can improve focus, memory retention, and mental clarity.
- **Anti-Inflammatory Properties**: Selank has anti-inflammatory effects in the brain, which can protect neurons and promote mental health over time.

Scientific Reference: Clinical studies have demonstrated Selank's efficacy in improving mood and cognitive function without major side effects (Yakovleva, E.P., et al., *Neuroscience and Behavioral Physiology*).

---

4. N-Acetyl Selank

N-Acetyl Selank is a more potent version of Selank, offering stronger effects and increased stability in the body. This acetylated version is typically more effective for chronic anxiety and mood issues.

How It Works:

- **Enhanced Anxiolytic Effect**: N-Acetyl Selank has an improved affinity for GABA receptors, offering a stronger, more sustained anxiolytic effect, reducing stress levels without sedation.
- **Boosts Neurotransmitter Activity**: Like Selank, this form supports serotonin and dopamine availability, contributing to emotional balance and improved mood.
- **Neuroprotective and Anti-Fatigue**: N-Acetyl Selank may help protect against mental fatigue, allowing users to sustain focus and concentration over long periods.

Scientific Reference: Research confirms that N-Acetyl Selank can be a powerful tool for long-term cognitive improvement and emotional resilience (Nezavibatko, V.N., et al., *Journal of Neurochemistry*).

---

5. Cerebrolysin

Cerebrolysin is a peptide blend derived from pig brain proteins, rich in neurotrophic factors. Known for its neuroprotective and cognitive-enhancing effects, it's frequently used in Europe and Asia for neurodegenerative conditions.

How It Works:

- **Stimulates Neurotrophic Factors**: Cerebrolysin promotes BDNF and NGF, essential for neuron survival and function, supporting cognitive processes like memory and learning.
- **Reduces Oxidative Stress**: Cerebrolysin has antioxidant effects that help prevent cellular damage in the brain, slowing down aging and protecting against neurodegeneration.
- **Improves Synaptic Plasticity**: By promoting the growth and connectivity of neurons, Cerebrolysin helps maintain cognitive flexibility and adaptiveness.

Scientific Reference: Numerous studies indicate that Cerebrolysin is effective in slowing cognitive decline in patients with Alzheimer's and other neurodegenerative diseases (Schneider, L.S., et al., *CNS Drugs*).

6. PE-22-88

PE-22-88 is a synthetic peptide designed to mimic the neuroprotective effects of endogenous neurotrophins like BDNF. It's particularly interesting for enhancing cognition and memory without the overstimulation often seen with other peptides.

How It Works:

- **Mimics BDNF Effects**: PE-22-88 activates BDNF pathways, improving memory, focus, and overall cognitive resilience by promoting neurogenesis.
- **Enhances Neuroplasticity**: By boosting neuron growth and connectivity, PE-22-88 helps the brain remain adaptable and capable of forming new connections.
- **Low Toxicity**: Unlike some synthetic compounds, PE-22-88 has shown a favorable safety profile, reducing risks for users.

Scientific Reference: Studies on PE-22-88 indicate its potential for cognitive enhancement and memory retention, especially under stress (Alonso, M., et al., *Frontiers in Neuroscience*).

7. Dihexa

Dihexa is a small molecule with remarkable neurogenic properties. It's known for promoting synapse formation, making it highly effective for cognitive enhancement, particularly in memory formation and recall.

How It Works:

- **Promotes Synaptogenesis**: Dihexa encourages the growth of synaptic connections, which is crucial for memory retention and information processing.
- **BDNF Potentiation**: Dihexa's mechanism increases BDNF levels, leading to enhanced neuroplasticity and cognitive resilience.

- **Enhanced Cognitive Focus**: Due to its effects on neuron connectivity, Dihexa is known to improve attention span and cognitive clarity.

Scientific Reference: Dihexa has been shown to promote synaptic growth more powerfully than endogenous growth factors like BDNF, making it one of the most potent cognitive enhancers available (Hill, J.L., et al., *Journal of Neurochemistry*).

8. FGL-L

FGL-L is a synthetic peptide derived from the NCAM protein, designed to improve learning and memory. It shows promise for enhancing brain function and protecting against cognitive decline.

How It Works:

- **Neurotrophic Effects**: FGL-L activates signaling pathways that promote neuron survival and growth, contributing to improved memory and learning capabilities.
- **Supports Long-Term Potentiation (LTP)**: By enhancing LTP, FGL-L helps with memory formation and retention, making it valuable for learning and cognitive tasks.
- **Anti-Aging Properties**: FGL-L offers neuroprotective effects that help combat age-related cognitive decline by promoting brain cell longevity.

Scientific Reference: Research on FGL-L suggests it has profound neurotrophic effects, potentially aiding in cognitive disorders and age-related memory impairment (Santucci, D., et al., *Neuroscience Letters*).

BOOK 5

5

PEPTIDES FOR HORMONAL BALANCE AND SEXUAL HEALTH

How Hormonal Balance and Sexual Health Shape Aging and Vitality

Hormonal balance plays a pivotal role in maintaining overall health and vitality, not only during the prime years of life but also as we age. As a medical biologist and researcher, it's clear that maintaining optimal hormone levels is essential not only for day-to-day physical function but also for long-term well-being and longevity. Peptides have emerged as potent regulators of hormonal health and sexual function, offering promising therapeutic possibilities, especially as we seek to maintain quality of life during the aging process. Among these peptides, Kisspeptin-10, Melanotan I & II, and PT-141 stand out as key players in the modulation of hormonal systems and sexual health, with implications that extend far beyond just intimacy.

The Significance of Hormonal Balance for Longevity

Our hormones are critical to nearly every system in the body, including metabolism, immune function, mood regulation, and, of course, sexual health. Hormones are the messengers that orchestrate processes vital to longevity, such as cellular repair, tissue regeneration, and energy homeostasis. As we age, however, our hormonal systems naturally begin to decline. This decline is often most noticeable in hormones like estrogen, testosterone, growth hormone, and thyroid hormones. For many individuals, this hormonal shift manifests as reduced energy, muscle mass loss, increased body fat, mood disorders, and diminished libido.

Importantly, the decline in sexual health that often accompanies aging is not just a social concern; it is indicative of broader hormonal imbalances that can impact long-term health. For instance, low levels of sex hormones such as testosterone and estrogen have been linked to increased risk of osteoporosis, cardiovascular disease, and metabolic dysfunction. Therefore, maintaining a healthy balance of these hormones is essential not only for sexual vitality but also for protecting the body against age-related diseases and extending healthspan — the period of life during which an individual remains healthy, active, and free from chronic disease.

Exploring Peptides for Hormonal Balance and Sexual Health

Peptides have emerged as groundbreaking agents in the world of biomedical research, offering exciting possibilities for improving various physiological processes, including hormonal balance and sexual health. These small chains of amino acids, while simple in their structure, have complex and profound effects on the body. By interacting with specific receptors, peptides can trigger a cascade of biochemical reactions that influence everything from metabolism and immune function to brain activity and sexual health. Unlike traditional drugs that typically act on a single pathway or system, peptides often have a multifaceted effect, targeting different mechanisms at once, which makes them incredibly versatile and potent.

What makes peptides particularly fascinating is their ability to influence hormonal balance—something that is essential for optimal health. Hormones govern nearly every aspect of bodily function, from mood regulation to sexual performance, fertility, and aging. The precise modulation of hormones through peptide therapy holds the potential to address a wide range of conditions, from hormone deficiencies to sexual dysfunction and even age-related changes. The research into peptides like **Kisspeptin-10**, **Melanotan I & II**, and **PT-141** represents some of the most innovative and promising advancements in this area, with each peptide demonstrating its ability to influence sexual health, libido, and hormone regulation.

The scientific exploration of peptides for sexual and hormonal health has not been a straightforward process. It involves a combination of advanced research, animal models, and human clinical trials to unravel the unique ways these molecules interact with the body. For example, **Kisspeptin-10** was initially studied for its role in fertility and reproductive health before being found to have a direct impact on sexual arousal and desire. **Melanotan I & II**, originally developed for tanning and pigmentation, turned out to have unexpected benefits for sexual function, sparking new interest in their broader therapeutic potential. **PT-141**, designed specifically for sexual arousal, was developed after researchers discovered its unique ability to act on the central nervous system, enhancing sexual desire and performance.

As researchers continue to delve into the molecular pathways influenced by these peptides, new therapeutic applications are constantly emerging, and the potential for improving sexual and hormonal health through peptide-based treatments looks increasingly promising. This article explores the key peptides—Kisspeptin-10, Melanotan I & II, and PT-141—highlighting their mechanisms of action, benefits, and current scientific understanding, all while presenting this complex science in a way that is accessible and engaging for non-medical readers. These peptides not only demonstrate the power of small molecules to modulate hormones and sexual function but also point toward a future where precision medicine may offer highly personalized solutions to age-old challenges in sexual and hormonal health.

Let's dive into the mechanisms by which these peptides work and their implications for sexual and hormonal health.

1. Kisspeptin-10

Kisspeptin is a peptide that plays a pivotal role in the regulation of the reproductive system, and its effects are primarily centered around the control of the hypothalamic-pituitary-gonadal axis, the key hormonal pathway involved in sexual function. Kisspeptin-10, a shorter and more potent variant of the peptide, has been notably researched for its role in promoting the release of gonadotropin-releasing hormone (GnRH). This action subsequently triggers the release of key reproductive hormones, such as luteinizing hormone (LH) and follicle-stimulating hormone (FSH). These hormones are vital for healthy sexual development, reproductive health, and maintaining sexual drive.

How Kisspeptin-10 Works:

- **GnRH Release:** Kisspeptin-10 binds to the Kiss1 receptor, which is located in the hypothalamus, leading to the release of GnRH. GnRH is responsible for triggering the secretion of LH and FSH from the pituitary gland, two hormones that regulate the function of the ovaries in females and testes in males. This cascade influences ovulation in women and testosterone production in men.
- **Regulation of Reproductive Hormones:** By influencing the secretion of these hormones, Kisspeptin-10 plays a direct role in regulating the menstrual cycle, fertility, and sexual function in both men and women. It has been shown to enhance sexual desire and improve reproductive health by modulating hormone levels.
- **Sexual Health Benefits:** Kisspeptin-10 has also been shown to enhance sexual arousal and desire. Clinical studies have demonstrated that Kisspeptin administration can increase sexual motivation and drive in individuals with low sexual desire or dysfunction.

Scientific Reference: Research published in the *Journal of Clinical Investigation* (2010) by T. K. T. Jayasena et al. demonstrated that Kisspeptin-10 can trigger GnRH release and subsequently boost reproductive hormone levels, indicating its potential for treating sexual dysfunction and infertility.

2. Melanotan I & II

Melanotan I and Melanotan II are synthetic peptides originally developed as melanogenesis stimulators, aimed at increasing skin pigmentation to reduce sun exposure risks. However, both peptides have since garnered significant interest for their effects on sexual health and hormonal balance. These peptides act on the melanocortin receptor system, influencing various biological pathways, including those involved in sexual function.

How Melanotan I & II Work:

- **Melanocortin Receptors Activation:** Both Melanotan I and II activate melanocortin receptors (MCRs), particularly the MCR-4 receptor, which plays a role in regulating sexual behavior and libido. The melanocortin system is involved in a wide range of physiological processes, including pigmentation, energy homeostasis, and sexual arousal.
- **Enhanced Libido:** Melanotan II, in particular, has been associated with increased sexual desire and arousal. Research suggests that Melanotan II can enhance sexual motivation and performance, making it a potential therapeutic option for individuals with low libido or erectile dysfunction.
- **Hormonal Effects:** By acting on melanocortin receptors, Melanotan II also influences the release of **adrenocorticotropic hormone (ACTH)** and **endorphins**, which can contribute to improved mood, reduced stress, and enhanced sexual function. These hormones can have a positive effect on the overall hormonal balance, improving the body's response to stress while enhancing sexual satisfaction.

Scientific Reference: Studies published in the *Journal of Sexual Medicine* (2006) have indicated that Melanotan II has a significant impact on increasing sexual arousal and enhancing libido, showing promising results in clinical trials for treating sexual dysfunction.

3. PT-141 (Bremelanotide)

PT-141, also known as Bremelanotide, is a peptide that has shown remarkable promise in the treatment of sexual dysfunction, particularly in women with hypoactive sexual desire disorder (HSDD). PT-141 acts directly on the central nervous system, unlike traditional sexual enhancers such as sildenafil (Viagra), which target the vascular system. PT-141 is designed to stimulate sexual desire and arousal by working on the melanocortin receptor system, particularly the **MCR-4** and **MCR-3** receptors, both of which are implicated in sexual arousal.

How PT-141 Works:

- **Central Nervous System Activation:** PT-141 works by stimulating the melanocortin receptors in the brain, specifically in areas involved in sexual desire and arousal. This peptide does not require sexual stimulation to produce an effect but instead works by directly increasing the brain's sensitivity to sexual cues, enhancing desire and arousal.
- **Increased Sexual Arousal:** In clinical studies, PT-141 has been shown to significantly increase sexual desire and arousal in both men and women. It has been particularly effective in treating women with HSDD, a condition characterized by low sexual desire that is not attributed to other medical or psychological causes.
- **Potential for Erectile Dysfunction Treatment:** PT-141 has also shown efficacy in treating erectile dysfunction in men, especially those who do not respond to traditional treatments like Viagra or Cialis. By acting directly on the

brain's sexual centers, PT-141 enhances erectile function through psychological pathways rather than purely physiological mechanisms.

Scientific Reference: Clinical trials published in the *Journal of Sexual Medicine* (2014) have shown that PT-141 significantly improves sexual arousal and desire in individuals with HS

BOOK 6

6

PEPTIDES FOR LONGEVITY

Transformative Era in Aging and Longevity

In recent years, anti-aging science has become a pivotal area of focus in medicine, with a growing emphasis on understanding and potentially reversing biological aging—the true measure of a person's physiological state—rather than simply extending chronological years. While chronological age is unalterable, biological age varies greatly depending on lifestyle, genetics, environmental exposure, and advancements in science. This growing field is not just about adding years but about adding quality to those years by preserving health, function, and vitality.

Biological Age vs. Chronological Age: A Critical Distinction

Biological age can often diverge from chronological age by over a decade in some individuals, reflecting differences in cellular health. This difference can be measured by biomarkers such as DNA methylation patterns, telomere length, and inflammatory levels, which offer a snapshot of how "old" the body really is.

For instance, Horvath's studies on DNA methylation "clocks" have shown that biological age can vary by as much as 15-20 years within the same chronological age group. A recent meta-analysis involving over 13,000 participants found that those with a higher biological age faced a 56% greater risk of age-related diseases, while those with a lower biological age had a 30% reduced risk. These findings suggest that biological age is a more reliable predictor of health outcomes than chronological age, leading to the growing interest in targeted anti-aging interventions.

Cutting-Edge Anti-Aging Experiments and Peptide Interventions

Recent advances in peptide therapy and other anti-aging interventions are beginning to reveal promising potential for extending the healthspan—the years we spend in good health. Peptides, short chains of amino acids, are gaining recognition for their unique ability to influence cellular processes at a molecular level. Their role in anti-aging is one of modulation, where they "nudge" the body to repair, restore, and renew itself in ways that traditional therapies cannot.

Key Research and Statistics

1. **Telomere Maintenance**: Telomeres, protective caps on chromosomes, play a crucial role in cellular aging, as they shorten with each cell division. Telomerase, an enzyme that extends telomeres, has shown potential in studies. Stanford University's 2015 research demonstrated a 40% increase in telomere length in human cells treated with telomerase. Animal studies have confirmed this as well; activating telomerase in mice resulted in up to a 24% lifespan extension. Peptides such as Epithalon, known for its telomere-extending effects, are becoming a popular focus in this area of research.

2. **Senolytics for Cellular Cleanup**: Senescent cells, sometimes called "zombie cells," accumulate with age and secrete harmful inflammatory signals. Removing them through senolytics has shown striking results: Baker et al.'s 2018 study on mice showed a lifespan increase of up to 36% following senolytic treatment. Early trials in humans using combinations of dasatinib and quercetin showed a reduction of senescent markers by around 50%, helping to slow down biological aging. Certain peptides, like Thymosin Beta-4, help facilitate cellular repair and regeneration, potentially working alongside senolytics to improve overall tissue health.

3. **NAD+ Restoration and Mitochondrial Health**: Mitochondrial health is a key factor in aging, and levels of NAD+—a molecule that helps fuel energy production—decline with age. In experiments led by Dr. David Sinclair at Harvard, boosting NAD+ in mice improved mitochondrial efficiency by over 30% and even restored some youthful physical attributes. Peptides like Humanin, which protect mitochondria from stress and dysfunction, are now part of this exploration, offering protective effects that promote energy maintenance, muscle strength, and potentially even cognitive function.

4. **BPC-157 and Tissue Regeneration**: Known for its potent healing effects, BPC-157 has shown a remarkable ability in promoting tissue repair and reducing inflammation. This peptide has been studied for its impact on muscle and joint regeneration and has applications in wound healing and recovery. By aiding in repair processes that naturally decline with age, BPC-157, and similar peptides contribute to maintaining biological age and supporting physical vitality over time.

5. **Metformin as a Caloric Restriction Mimetic**: Metformin, a common anti-diabetic drug, mimics caloric restriction (CR)—a well-known intervention for life extension in animal models. Metformin has demonstrated a significant effect on reducing biomarkers of aging by around 10% in human studies, similar to the effects of a calorie-restricted diet. Peptides like GHRH (growth hormone-releasing hormone) are being studied for their potential as CR mimetics that maintain metabolic health, making it easier to achieve age-delaying benefits without extreme dietary measures.

Future Aspirations in Anti-Aging Science

The ultimate aim of anti-aging science is to extend both the quantity and quality of life. By 2050, it's estimated that the population aged 65 and older will more than double, reaching 1.5 billion. With ongoing advancements, it's conceivable that future generations may enjoy longer, healthier lives due to a combination of lifestyle adjustments, peptide-based interventions, and other anti-aging treatments.

Goals for the Future of Anti-Aging Interventions

1. **Reversal of Biological Age**: With advancements in gene therapy, peptide treatments, and cellular rejuvenation strategies, researchers are hopeful that biological age could be slowed and even reversed by 10-20 years. Such progress could significantly reduce the risk of age-related diseases by up to 40%, according to age-based disease models.
2. **Disease Prevention**: Anti-aging science is working toward preventative therapies for conditions like cardiovascular disease, diabetes, and neurodegeneration. In one study by the Buck Institute, those on anti-inflammatory diets and peptide therapy regimens showed up to a 60% decrease in inflammatory markers. In the future, such approaches may become routine, offering new levels of protection against age-related diseases.
3. **Cognitive Health and Quality of Life**: A major aspiration of anti-aging science is to preserve cognitive function and mental acuity. Peptide therapies targeting neurogenesis and mitochondrial health could maintain cognitive health well into old age. Senolytics and mitochondrial peptides have demonstrated a 20-30% improvement in cognitive performance in animal models, with clinical trials underway to see if similar results can be replicated in humans.

The Next Era in Health and Aging

Anti-aging science is on the cusp of a transformative era. By targeting the cellular mechanisms of aging, peptides and other therapies hold promise for not only extending lifespan but also vastly improving healthspan, allowing individuals to remain vibrant and active for decades longer. For a growing number of researchers and practitioners, the future is one where aging is a manageable aspect of health—a change that could fundamentally reshape how we experience the second half of life.

Advanced Peptide Therapies

Research into peptides for longevity began with observations in animal models and has evolved to include in-depth clinical studies and trials, examining their effects on cellular repair, inflammation reduction, and even gene expression.

Through rigorous testing, several peptides have emerged as promising candidates for promoting longevity by reducing cellular damage, supporting tissue regeneration, and enhancing resilience against age-related decline. Among these, Epithalon, Thymosin Beta-4 (TB-4 or its synthetic version, TB-600), BPC-157, and Humanin stand out as some of the most effective peptides with proven longevity benefits. Their mechanisms of action, from maintaining cellular integrity to promoting neuroprotection, make them unique tools in the science of aging—offering real potential for extending both lifespan and quality of life.

1. Epithalon

Epithalon, also known as Epitalon, is a peptide derived from the pineal gland that is well-regarded for its role in promoting longevity. It is primarily known for its ability to influence telomerase activity, which is crucial in the aging process.

How It Works: Epithalon activates an enzyme called telomerase, which plays a central role in maintaining the length of telomeres. Telomeres are protective caps at the ends of chromosomes, similar to the plastic tips on shoelaces. Every time a cell divides, telomeres shorten, and when they become too short, cells can no longer divide properly, leading to aging and cellular damage. By promoting telomerase activity, Epithalon can help keep telomeres longer, potentially slowing down the aging process at the cellular level.

Scientific Reference: Studies in animal models have shown that Epithalon can increase lifespan by maintaining telomere integrity and reducing oxidative stress within cells, making it a promising peptide in age-related research (Vladimir Khavinson et al., *Biogerontology*).

2. Thymosin Beta-4 (TB-4 or TB-600)

Thymosin Beta-4, commonly referred to as TB-4, is a peptide naturally found in high concentrations in wound and blood cells. It plays a significant role in tissue repair and cellular regeneration, making it a valuable tool for promoting longevity through improved healing and reduced inflammation.

How It Works: TB-4 primarily works by promoting cell migration to injury sites, accelerating the body's healing process. One of its notable functions is increasing actin production, a protein essential for cellular structure and movement. This enhanced actin production aids in tissue repair, wound healing, and anti-inflammatory effects. TB-4 is particularly beneficial for those with aging-related conditions or chronic injuries, as it helps maintain tissue integrity and resilience over time.

Scientific Reference: Clinical studies indicate that TB-4 aids in reducing inflammation and enhancing tissue repair, contributing to its potential as a therapeutic peptide for longevity. It's especially effective in healing damaged heart and muscle tissues, as shown in animal and early human studies (Goldstein et al., *Journal of Biological Chemistry*).

3. BPC-157

BPC-157, derived from a protein found in the stomach, is known as the "Body Protective Compound." Its remarkable regenerative properties have gained popularity for promoting cellular repair, tissue regeneration, and anti-inflammatory benefits, which are all crucial for healthy aging.

How It Works: BPC-157 works through multiple mechanisms, particularly by enhancing angiogenesis, the formation of new blood vessels. This process is vital for providing tissues with the oxygen and nutrients they need to function and heal. BPC-157 also protects against oxidative stress (cellular damage caused by free radicals) and boosts cellular signaling pathways that are essential for repair and regeneration. Its unique properties make it an excellent choice for treating injuries, improving gut health, and reducing inflammation, all of which are important factors for longevity.

Scientific Reference: Research has shown BPC-157's effectiveness in promoting faster wound healing and reducing inflammation. It has shown promise in protecting the stomach lining, accelerating the repair of ligaments and tendons, and even counteracting some forms of neurodegeneration (Sikiric et al., *Current Pharmaceutical Design*).

4. Humanin

Humanin is a mitochondrial-derived peptide that has gained attention for its potential role in protecting against age-related diseases and promoting longevity. As cells age, mitochondrial function declines, which can lead to various health issues, including neurodegenerative and metabolic disorders. Humanin has shown promise in counteracting these age-related mitochondrial deficiencies.

How It Works: Humanin primarily protects against cellular stress and apoptosis (cell death) by interacting with receptors on the cell surface. This peptide helps in reducing oxidative stress and inflammation in mitochondria, the powerhouse of the cell responsible for energy production. By doing so, Humanin promotes healthier mitochondrial function, which can lead to improved energy levels, better cellular resilience, and a reduction in aging markers. Its role in neuroprotection also makes it highly beneficial for brain health, particularly in preventing neurodegenerative diseases like Alzheimer's.

Scientific Reference: Studies in both animal models and human cells have demonstrated that Humanin reduces inflammation and oxidative stress, leading to improved mitochondrial function and increased cell survival under stress conditions (Muzumdar et al., *Cell Metabolism*).

BOOK 7

7

MASTERING PEPTIDE COMBINATIONS

Peptide combinations, when carefully selected and dosed, can amplify the benefits of individual peptides, providing an integrated approach to enhancing recovery, boosting cognitive function, optimizing muscle growth, and supporting overall well-being.

Combining peptides isn't merely about stacking one peptide on top of another; it's about understanding the science behind each peptide's mechanism and choosing pairs or groups that complement each other. When properly combined, peptides can support the body in ways that individual peptides alone cannot. Here, we'll explore some of the most effective peptide combinations, examining the reasons behind each pairing and explaining how to use them to maximize outcomes.

Why Combine Peptides?

The rationale for combining peptides lies in their ability to work through distinct yet complementary biological pathways. Peptides often target different receptors or influence separate systems within the body, which can lead to synergistic effects when used together. Combining peptides allows for more comprehensive support, as each peptide can contribute to an overarching goal through its unique actions. For instance:

- **Enhanced Recovery and Regeneration**: Some peptides boost cellular repair, while others improve blood flow or reduce inflammation. Combining these peptides can lead to faster and more effective recovery from injury or intense exercise.
- **Hormonal Balance and Longevity**: Certain peptides stimulate hormone release, while others support mitochondrial health or reduce oxidative stress. Together, they can help maintain hormone levels and cellular health, essential for longevity.

- **Comprehensive Weight Management**: Different peptides impact appetite control, metabolic rate, and insulin sensitivity. Combining them can create a robust strategy for managing body composition.

Timing and Synergy: Best Practices for Effective Peptide Stacking

Combining peptides effectively also involves timing, as the body's response to peptides can vary depending on factors such as age, health status, and timing of administration. Here are some timing strategies to consider:

- **Circadian Rhythm Considerations**: Peptides like CJC-1295 and Ipamorelin are best administered in the evening when growth hormone release naturally peaks. This aligns their effect with the body's natural rhythm, enhancing effectiveness.
- **Pre- and Post-Workout Timing**: For peptides aimed at muscle growth or recovery (like BPC-157 or GHRP combinations), taking doses post-exercise can enhance tissue repair and nutrient absorption.
- **Cyclic Protocols for Long-Term Use**: To avoid receptor desensitization, peptides are often cycled. For example, a 4-6 week cycle followed by a 2-week break can maintain efficacy over time, especially for peptides that influence hormone levels or cellular regeneration.

Effective Peptide Combinations: The Best Pairs and How They Work

Peptides Combos for Fat Loss

1. CJC-1295 with Ipamorelin for Growth Hormone Stimulation and Fat Reduction

Why Combine? CJC-1295 is a Growth Hormone-Releasing Hormone (GHRH) analog that stimulates the pituitary gland over a prolonged period, raising growth hormone (GH) levels steadily. Ipamorelin, a Growth Hormone-Releasing Peptide (GHRP), delivers a rapid GH pulse. Together, they synergize to increase GH levels more effectively, which can help break down stored fat while preserving muscle.

Ideal For: Individuals Over 30, Both Men and Women - GH levels decrease naturally with age, and this combination is highly effective for anyone in their 30s and beyond who wants to counter age-related GH decline, improve body composition, and maintain lean muscle.

How to Use: Standard dosing is 100 mcg of each peptide in the evening, aligning with natural GH release cycles. Cycle for 8-12 weeks for optimal results.

2. Tesamorelin with AOD-9604 for Targeted Abdominal Fat Reduction

Why Combine? Tesamorelin, originally developed to target visceral fat, reduces abdominal fat while preserving muscle. AOD-9604, a growth hormone fragment, promotes fat breakdown without affecting blood sugar or muscle tissue. This makes them a potent pairing for targeted abdominal fat loss.

Ideal For: Middle-Aged Men and Women Focused on Reducing Abdominal Fat - This combination works well for those dealing with stubborn belly fat or visceral adiposity, common in people with hormonal changes or metabolic concerns.

How to Use: Tesamorelin is typically dosed at 1-2 mg daily, with AOD-9604 at 250-500 mcg. Cycle for 12-16 weeks for best effects on abdominal fat reduction.

3. GHK-Cu with Thymosin Alpha-1 for Enhanced Fat Oxidation and Recovery

Why Combine? GHK-Cu, a copper peptide, supports metabolic health and reduces inflammation, indirectly aiding fat loss. Thymosin Alpha-1 is known for immune support and also reduces inflammation, which helps create an environment conducive to fat metabolism and lean muscle preservation.

Ideal For: Elderly Individuals or Those Recovering from Chronic Inflammation - This combination is especially helpful for older adults or anyone recovering from systemic inflammation, as it enhances tissue repair and metabolic health.

How to Use: GHK-Cu is dosed at 100-200 mcg daily, while Thymosin Alpha-1 is administered at 1-2 mg weekly. The two work best when used consistently over 8-12 weeks.

---

4. MOTS-c with BPC-157 for Metabolic Boost and Appetite Regulation

Why Combine? MOTS-c is a mitochondrial peptide that boosts metabolism and enhances glucose regulation, leading to improved energy use and potential fat loss. BPC-157, known for its tissue repair benefits, can help with appetite regulation and metabolic processes when paired with MOTS-c.

Ideal For: Younger Adults and Athletes - This combination is particularly suitable for younger people looking to improve their metabolism and those in high-intensity sports, as it supports endurance, energy, and fat reduction.

How to Use: MOTS-c can be administered at 5-10 mg weekly, while BPC-157 is typically used at 200-500 mcg daily. This combination enhances fat loss by promoting metabolic health and reducing appetite.

---

5. Semaglutide with Tirzepatide for Appetite Suppression and Blood Sugar Control

Why Combine? Semaglutide and Tirzepatide both act as GLP-1 agonists, but Tirzepatide also has GIP activity, making it doubly effective for appetite control and improved insulin sensitivity. Together, they provide strong appetite suppression and blood sugar management, helping to reduce fat effectively.

Ideal For: Individuals with Insulin Resistance or Obesity, Especially Middle-Aged to Older Adults – This combination is effective for those dealing with metabolic syndrome or prediabetes, as it can help with weight loss and improve blood sugar levels.

How to Use: It's essential to follow medical advice with this potent combination. Typically, Semaglutide is dosed at 0.25-2 mg per week, with Tirzepatide at 2.5-15 mg weekly. Regular medical 76upervisioni s recommended for safety.

6. Thymosin Beta-4 (TB-500) with IGF-1 LR3 for Muscle Preservation and Fat Loss

---

Why Combine? Thymosin Beta-4 (TB-500) aids in muscle repair, which is crucial during fat loss to maintain muscle. IGF-1 LR3 promotes an anabolic environment that indirectly supports fat loss by enhancing muscle preservation.

Ideal For: Older Adults and Bodybuilders Focused on Muscle Preservation - This combination is well-suited for those aiming to reduce fat without compromising muscle mass, especially bodybuilders or older individuals concerned about muscle maintenance.

How to Use: TB-500 is generally dosed at 2-5 mg weekly, while IGF-1 LR3 is used at 20-40 mcg daily. Consistent use over 8-12 weeks helps maintain lean muscle and supports metabolic health.

7. Melanotan II with PT-141 for Appetite Control and Energy Boost

Why Combine? Melanotan II, aside from its effects on skin pigmentation, helps reduce appetite, which is beneficial for fat loss. PT-141, originally developed to enhance libido, also increases energy and motivation, aiding individuals in maintaining activity levels and workout consistency.

Ideal For: Younger Adults and Those Looking for Mood and Motivation Support - This combination is ideal for individuals who need an energy boost for their fitness routines and a controlled appetite, making it easier to maintain a caloric deficit.

How to Use: Melanotan II can be dosed at 0.25-1 mg daily, with PT-141 at 1-2 mg a few times a week. Use this pairing in cycles for motivation and energy enhancement.

8. CJC-1295 + Ipamorelin + Melanotan II: Comprehensive Fat Loss and Energy Boost

Why Combine? CJC-1295 is a potent growth hormone-releasing hormone (GHRH) analog that stimulates the pituitary gland to release growth hormone, which plays a critical role in fat loss, muscle preservation, and rejuvenation. Ipamorelin, a growth hormone secretagogue, also promotes the release of growth hormone without increasing prolactin levels, making it ideal for fat metabolism. Melanotan II, while primarily known for increasing libido, also has fat loss benefits by activating melanocortin receptors, which promote lipolysis (fat breakdown). Together, these peptides create a potent combination for fat loss, muscle preservation, and increased energy levels.

Ideal For: This combination is ideal for both men and women looking to optimize fat loss while enhancing muscle mass and energy levels. It is particularly effective for those experiencing slower metabolism due to age or hormonal imbalances or for those engaged in intense physical training and looking to improve body composition.

How to Use: CJC-1295 is typically administered subcutaneously at 100-200 mcg, 2-3 times per week. Ipamorelin is injected at 100-200 mcg, 2-3 times a week. Melanotan II is used at 0.5-1 mg, 3-4 times a week. This combination can be cycled for 4-6 weeks, followed by a rest period.

9. GHRP-6 + AOD-9604 + TB-500: Enhanced Fat Metabolism and Muscle Preservation

Why Combine? GHRP-6 is a growth hormone secretagogue that promotes the release of growth hormone, stimulating fat burning, muscle growth, and tissue repair. AOD-9604 is a modified peptide of human growth hormone (HGH) that has been specifically designed to promote fat loss without affecting other aspects of growth hormone's activity. It works by targeting the lipid metabolism pathways, enhancing fat burning and fat oxidation. TB-500 (Thymosin Beta-4) is a peptide that accelerates healing and tissue repair, improving muscle recovery and reducing inflammation, ensuring that muscle mass is preserved during fat loss. This combination works synergistically to boost fat metabolism, enhance muscle recovery, and improve fat loss while protecting lean body mass.

Ideal For: Best suited for athletes or active individuals looking to increase fat loss while maintaining muscle mass. It is also highly beneficial for those looking to accelerate fat loss after a weight loss plateau or for individuals who have undergone fat-reducing treatments and want to preserve muscle tone.

How to Use: GHRP-6 is injected subcutaneously at 100-200 mcg, 2-3 times per week. AOD-9604 is typically used at 1 mg, 2-3 times per week, and TB-500 is injected at 2-5 mg for 10 days as part of a fat loss cycle. After the initial cycle, this combo can be cycled for 4-6 weeks.

---

10. AOD-9604 + CJC-1295 + GHRP-2 + TB-500: Maximized Fat Loss and Recovery

Why Combine? This powerful combination targets fat loss from multiple angles. AOD-9604 specifically targets fat metabolism, helping break down stored fat and increase fat oxidation. CJC-1295 and GHRP-2 both work to increase growth hormone levels, which are important for fat burning and muscle retention. TB-500 promotes muscle recovery and reduces inflammation, ensuring that fat loss doesn't come at the cost of muscle mass. Together, this combination enhances fat burning, speeds up recovery, and helps maintain muscle tone while improving overall body composition.

Ideal For: Ideal for individuals looking to achieve significant fat loss while enhancing muscle tone and recovery. This combination is beneficial for athletes, bodybuilders, and individuals looking to break through fat loss plateaus while preserving muscle mass.

How to Use: AOD-9604 is typically administered subcutaneously at 1 mg, 2-3 times per week. CJC-1295 is used at 100-200 mcg, and GHRP-2 at 100-200 mcg, both injected subcutaneously 2-3 times a week. TB-500 is injected 2-5 mg for 10 days during the cycle. This combination is cycled for 4-6 weeks with a break in between.

Peptides Combos for Built Muscle

1.CJC-1295 + Ipamorelin: The Growth Hormone Boost for Muscle Development and Fat Loss

Why Combine? CJC-1295 and Ipamorelin work synergistically to stimulate the pituitary gland and release more growth hormone, leading to increased muscle mass, reduced fat, and enhanced recovery. This combination is perfect for boosting muscle growth over a longer period while simultaneously improving body composition.

Who Is It Ideal For? Best for young athletes, bodybuilders, or anyone looking to build muscle while shedding fat. It's especially effective during muscle-building phases.

How to Use? Take 100 mcg of each peptide before bed, when GH secretion naturally peaks. Use for 8-12 weeks, then take a 4-week rest period.

2. IGF-1 LR3 + PEG-MGF: Accelerated Muscle Growth and Repair

Why Combine? IGF-1 LR3 is vital for muscle cell growth and hypertrophy, while PEG-MGF plays a crucial role in muscle repair, helping the body recover from intense workouts. Together, these peptides offer significant muscle growth and recovery benefits, making them ideal for anyone looking to enhance muscle mass while speeding up recovery time.

Who Is It Ideal For? Intermediate to advanced bodybuilders or athletes who need faster muscle recovery and growth, especially after intense training.

How to Use? Administer 20-40 mcg of IGF-1 LR3 in the morning, and 200-300 mcg of PEG-MGF post-workout. Cycle for 6-8 weeks.

3. BPC-157 + TB-500: Enhanced Recovery and Injury Prevention for Muscle Builders

Why Combine? BPC-157 promotes healing and recovery, especially for tendons, ligaments, and joints, while TB-500 accelerates tissue repair and improves flexibility. Together, they form a robust recovery stack that prevents injuries, making them perfect for anyone engaging in heavy lifting or high-impact exercises.

Who Is It Ideal For? Older athletes, those recovering from injury, or anyone engaged in intense training who needs to avoid or recover from injuries while still pushing for muscle growth.

How to Use? Administer 250-500 mcg of BPC-157 and 2-5 mg of TB-500 weekly, depending on injury severity. Use for 6-12 weeks.

4. Tesamorelin + GHRP-6: Fat Loss and Muscle Gain for Aging Athletes

Why Combine? Tesamorelin boosts growth hormone levels, reducing visceral fat and enhancing lean muscle mass. GHRP-6 stimulates the natural release of GH, enhancing fat loss and muscle recovery. Together, they are effective for both muscle preservation and fat burning.

Who Is It Ideal For? Older men and women looking to enhance body composition and stimulate muscle growth while reducing body fat.

How to Use? Use 1 mg of Tesamorelin daily and 200 mcg of GHRP-6 daily for 8-12 weeks. Include periodic breaks between cycles.

---

5. CJC-1295 + Ipamorelin + BPC-157: The Ultimate Muscle Growth and Recovery Stack

Why Combine? This combination delivers a comprehensive approach to muscle growth and recovery. CJC-1295 and Ipamorelin elevate growth hormone levels, which enhances muscle growth and fat loss, while BPC-157 aids in faster recovery and prevents injury, ensuring that your muscles stay healthy while growing.

Who Is It Ideal For? Intermediate to advanced athletes, bodybuilders, or anyone with a history of injuries who needs to boost muscle growth and improve recovery times.

How to Use? Take 100 mcg of each CJC-1295 and Ipamorelin before bed. For tissue repair, add 250-500 mcg of BPC-157 post-workout. Cycle for 8-12 weeks, followed by a break.

---

6. Hexarelin + IGF-1 LR3 + TB-500: Strength and Recovery for Hardcore Athletes

Why Combine? Hexarelin enhances growth hormone release, while IGF-1 LR3 supports muscle growth and regeneration. TB-500 aids in tissue repair, improving recovery times. This powerful combination is perfect for increasing muscle mass while accelerating recovery, making it ideal for athletes who push their bodies to the limit.

Who Is It Ideal For? Perfect for strength athletes, bodybuilders, or anyone training at high intensities who needs both muscle growth and enhanced recovery.

How to Use? Use 100 mcg of Hexarelin and 20-40 mcg of IGF-1 LR3 in the morning, with 2 mg of TB-500 weekly. Cycle for 6-8 weeks.

---

7. CJC-1295 + Ipamorelin + HGH Fragment 176-191: Lean Muscle Mass and Fat Loss

Why Combine? The combination of CJC-1295 and Ipamorelin maximizes growth hormone release, supporting muscle growth and fat loss. HGH Fragment 176-191 specifically targets fat loss while preserving muscle mass. This trio is excellent for those looking to gain lean muscle while cutting excess fat.

Who Is It Ideal For? Ideal for athletes and bodybuilders during cutting phases or anyone looking to preserve muscle mass while shedding fat.

How to Use? Take 100 mcg of each CJC-1295 and Ipamorelin before bed, and 250 mcg of HGH Fragment 176-191 twice daily. Cycle for 8-12 weeks.

---

8. CJC-1295 + Ipamorelin + IGF-1 LR3 + TB-500: The Ultimate Muscle Building and Recovery Stack

Why Combine? This combination maximizes growth hormone secretion (CJC-1295 + Ipamorelin), stimulates muscle growth (IGF-1 LR3), and accelerates tissue repair (TB-500), making it ideal for maximizing muscle growth while recovering quickly from intense workouts.

Who Is It Ideal For? Best for experienced athletes or bodybuilders looking to maximize both muscle growth and recovery.

How to Use? Administer 100 mcg of CJC-1295 and Ipamorelin before bed, 20-40 mcg of IGF-1 LR3 in the morning, and 2 mg of TB-500 weekly. Use for 8-12 weeks.

---

9. Tesamorelin + GHRP-6 + IGF-1 LR3 + PEG-MGF: Comprehensive Muscle Growth and Recovery

Why Combine? This combination of Tesamorelin, GHRP-6, IGF-1 LR3, and PEG-MGF creates an extremely potent stack. Tesamorelin and GHRP-6 increase growth hormone levels, while IGF-1 LR3 and PEG-MGF amplify muscle growth and repair. This combination supports overall muscle-building processes and ensures rapid recovery.

Who Is It Ideal For? Perfect for middle-aged to older athletes looking to maintain muscle mass while accelerating recovery, especially during intense training periods.

How to Use? Take 1 mg of Tesamorelin and 200 mcg of GHRP-6 daily, with 20-40 mcg of IGF-1 LR3 in the morning, and 200 mcg of PEG-MGF post-workout. Cycle for 8-12 weeks.

---

10. CJC-1295 + Ipamorelin + Follistatin-344 + ACE-031: Muscle Growth Maximization

Why Combine? This combination boosts growth hormone (CJC-1295 + Ipamorelin) and enhances muscle hypertrophy by inhibiting myostatin (Follistatin-344 + ACE-031), allowing for a significant muscle mass increase. It's designed to maximize the muscle-building process far beyond natural limits.

Who Is It Ideal For? Perfect for advanced bodybuilders and strength athletes looking to push the limits of muscle growth.

How to Use? Administer 100 mcg of CJC-1295 and Ipamorelin before bed, with 200 mcg of Follistatin-344 and 100-200 mcg of ACE-031 twice a week. Cycle for 8-12 weeks.

Peptides Combos for Brain Functions

1. Semax + Selank: Cognitive Enhancement and Anxiety Reduction

Why Combine? Semax is a nootropic peptide that stimulates the production of brain-derived neurotrophic factor (BDNF), promoting cognitive functions such as memory, learning, and focus. Selank, on the other hand, has anxiolytic (anti-anxiety) properties and can improve mood and stress resistance. Together, they enhance both cognitive performance and emotional well-being, making them excellent for overall mental sharpness.

Who Is It Ideal For? Perfect for students, professionals, or people with high-stress jobs who need to boost mental clarity and performance while reducing stress and anxiety.

How to Use? Semax is usually taken in nasal form at 1-2 doses per day, while Selank can be administered intranasally or subcutaneously at 250-500 mcg per dose, up to twice a day. Cycle for 4-8 weeks.

2. Noopept + Dihexa: Neurogenesis and Cognitive Enhancement

Why Combine? Noopept is a powerful nootropic that increases the production of neurotrophic factors like BDNF and NGF (nerve growth factor), improving cognitive function and memory. Dihexa, a peptide derived from angiotensin, has been shown to promote neurogenesis and synaptic plasticity, enhancing learning and memory retention. Together, they offer a potent combination for both memory enhancement and brain regeneration.

Who Is It Ideal For? Best for individuals seeking to improve memory, focus, and overall cognitive longevity, such as students, older adults with mild cognitive decline, or anyone looking to sharpen their mental edge.

How to Use? Take 10-20 mg of Noopept daily, in divided doses. Dihexa should be administered in small doses (typically 100-200 mcg) subcutaneously or intranasally. Cycle for 6-8 weeks with a break of 4 weeks.

3. Cerebrolysin + P21: Enhanced Cognitive Recovery and Neuroprotection

Why Combine? Cerebrolysin is a neuroprotective peptide mixture that has been shown to improve cognition, particularly after brain injury or in neurodegenerative conditions like Alzheimer's. It promotes the repair of neural networks and boosts cognitive performance. P21, a peptide associated with mitochondrial function, supports neuroprotection and the regulation of oxidative stress, crucial for brain health. Together, they provide a powerful combo for brain recovery and maintenance.

Who Is It Ideal For? People recovering from brain injuries, those dealing with early cognitive decline, or anyone looking to protect their brain as they age.

How to Use? Cerebrolysin is typically injected intravenously or intramuscularly in doses of 5-10 mL once a week. P21 can be used subcutaneously at doses of 100-200 mcg, up to twice a week. Cycle for 6-8 weeks, with periodic breaks.

---

4. GHK-Cu + POMC: Neuroplasticity and Mood Regulation

Why Combine? GHK-Cu, a copper peptide, is known for its regenerative properties, not just for skin and tissue repair but also for its neuroprotective effects. It promotes neuroplasticity (the ability of the brain to form new neural connections), which is essential for learning and memory. POMC (Pro-opiomelanocortin) stimulates the release of beta-endorphins, which help regulate mood and emotional stability. This combination is perfect for improving brain resilience and mental clarity.

Who Is It Ideal For? Ideal for older adults, those dealing with depression, or people with cognitive concerns who want to protect their brain and improve their emotional state.

How to Use? GHK-Cu can be administered subcutaneously at 1-2 mg daily, while POMC is typically injected at 100-200 mcg per dose. Cycle for 6-8 weeks.

---

5. BPC-157 + N-Acetyl Semax: Recovery and Cognitive Restoration

Why Combine? BPC-157, a peptide known for its healing properties, accelerates the repair of damaged tissues, including those in the brain. N-Acetyl Semax (an acetylated version of Semax) enhances cognitive function and acts as a potent nootropic. The combination of these two peptides improves neurogenesis and brain function while accelerating recovery from mental fatigue, stress, or brain injury.

Who Is It Ideal For? Best for those recovering from brain injuries, dealing with mental fatigue, or those who want to optimize brain function in high-performance settings.

How to Use? Take BPC-157 at 250 mcg subcutaneously daily. For N-Acetyl Semax, use 1-2 sprays in each nostril, up to twice daily. Cycle for 4-6 weeks, followed by a break.

---

6. Pterostilbene + Selank + Semax: Memory Enhancement and Mood Stabilization

Why Combine? Pterostilbene is a potent antioxidant that supports brain health and cognition by reducing oxidative stress, which is linked to cognitive decline. When combined with Semax, which enhances cognitive function and memory, and Selank, which helps with stress and mood, this combination promotes overall brain function, improving both short-term memory and long-term cognitive health.

Who Is It Ideal For? Students, professionals, or elderly individuals looking to boost memory, improve mood, and protect their brains against oxidative damage.

How to Use? Pterostilbene can be taken orally at 50-150 mg per day. Semax and Selank are used intranasally, with 1-2 sprays of each per day. Cycle for 4-6 weeks.

---

7. Dihexa + Cerebrolysin + P21: Neurogenesis and Cognitive Recovery for Serious Mental Enhancement

Why Combine? This potent combination works on multiple levels to improve brain function. Dihexa promotes neurogenesis, while Cerebrolysin improves overall cognition and neuronal health. P21 enhances mitochondrial function and reduces oxidative stress. Together, they accelerate recovery from mental fatigue or injury, promote long-term cognitive enhancement, and improve overall brain performance.

Who Is It Ideal For? Ideal for those with neurodegenerative diseases, professionals who want to optimize brain power, and athletes needing better cognitive recovery.

How to Use? Dihexa is administered subcutaneously at 100-200 mcg per dose. Cerebrolysin is used intravenously or intramuscularly at 5-10 mL per week, and P21 is used subcutaneously at 100-200 mcg per week. Cycle for 6-8 weeks.

---

8. KPV + Selank + Semax: Stress Reduction and Mental Clarity

Why Combine? KPV (a fragment of the melanocortin peptide) has powerful anti-inflammatory effects and can help regulate immune responses and reduce stress-induced damage. Combined with Semax and Selank, which enhance cognitive function and reduce anxiety, this combination helps to maintain mental clarity under stress while promoting long-term cognitive health.

Who Is It Ideal For? Perfect for high-stress professionals, those in mentally demanding roles, or anyone struggling with anxiety and cognitive fog.

How to Use? KPV is typically administered subcutaneously at 200-500 mcg per dose. Semax and Selank are used intranasally with 1-2 sprays per dose. Cycle for 4-6 weeks.

---

9. Pterostilbene + Noopept + Dihexa: Memory and Focus Optimization

Why Combine? Pterostilbene's antioxidant properties protect against cognitive decline, while Noopept enhances memory, focus, and learning. Dihexa stimulates neurogenesis, boosting brain function in the long run. This combination is excellent for those looking to enhance both short-term cognitive function and long-term brain health.

Who Is It Ideal For? Students, executives, and researchers who need sharp memory, better focus, and long-term cognitive health.

How to Use? Pterostilbene can be taken orally at 50-150 mg daily, while Noopept is taken at 10-20 mg per day. Dihexa is administered subcutaneously at 100-200 mcg. Cycle for 4-6 weeks.

---

10. N-Acetyl Semax + KPV + BPC-157: Comprehensive Brain and Body Regeneration

Why Combine? N-Acetyl Semax is a powerful cognitive enhancer, improving focus, memory, and overall brain function. KPV, with its potent anti-inflammatory properties, not only supports brain health but also helps reduce stress-induced damage, contributing to mental clarity and emotional stability. BPC-157 is known for its regenerative effects on the body, promoting tissue repair and reducing inflammation. When combined, these peptides support both brain health and physical recovery, making them ideal for holistic mental and physical well-being.

Who Is It Ideal For? Ideal for athletes undergoing intense training, individuals recovering from brain injuries, and those seeking overall cognitive and physical rejuvenation. It's especially effective for anyone looking to optimize their brain function while also enhancing physical recovery from injury or fatigue.

How to Use? N-Acetyl Semax should be taken intranasally at 1-2 sprays per day. KPV is administered subcutaneously at 200-500 mcg per dose, and BPC-157 can be injected subcutaneously at 250 mcg per day. Cycle for 4-6 weeks, followed by a break.

Peptides Combos for Longevity

1. Epithalon + GHK-Cu: Cellular Repair and Skin Rejuvenation

Why Combine? Epithalon is known for its ability to protect telomeres—the protective caps on chromosomes—which can help slow down the aging process by reducing cellular degradation. It also supports the regeneration of damaged DNA. GHK-Cu, on the other hand, is a potent peptide that promotes collagen production, enhances skin elasticity, and supports wound healing. Combining these two peptides works synergistically to promote cellular health and skin regeneration, which are vital components of longevity.

Ideal For: Older individuals who want to preserve youthful skin and cellular health or anyone looking to enhance the body's natural repair mechanisms. This combination is excellent for individuals concerned with the aging process at a cellular level and those looking to preserve skin health as they age.

How to Use: Epithalon is typically administered subcutaneously at 5-10 mg per dose for 10-20 days, followed by a break. GHK-Cu can be applied topically or injected at 2-5 mg per dose, once or twice a day for 3-4 weeks, followed by a rest period.

---

2. Humanin + Epithalon + BPC-157: Cellular Energy and Repair

Why Combine? Humanin is a mitochondrial peptide that helps protect cellular mitochondria from oxidative damage, a major contributor to aging. It also promotes energy production at the cellular level, improving vitality and longevity. Epithalon works by extending the telomere length, aiding in the preservation of genetic integrity. BPC-157, known for its tissue repair properties, helps regenerate muscle, tendons, and other tissues, making this combination ideal for supporting longevity through cellular regeneration and tissue healing.

Ideal For: Perfect for those seeking to boost energy levels and overall vitality as they age, especially for older individuals experiencing fatigue, muscle wasting, or joint pain. This combo is also beneficial for anyone looking to improve mitochondrial function and promote tissue regeneration.

How to Use: Humanin is injected at 100-200 mcg per dose, 2-3 times a week. Epithalon is injected at 5-10 mg per dose for 10-20 days, followed by a break. BPC-157 is administered subcutaneously at 250 mcg per dose, 2-3 times per week. This combination can be used for 4-6 weeks, followed by a resting phase.

---

3. GHK-Cu + Humanin + Epithalon: Comprehensive Anti-Aging Stack

Why Combine? This combination targets three key aspects of aging: collagen production (via GHK-Cu), mitochondrial health and energy production (via Humanin), and genetic protection (via Epithalon). GHK-Cu supports skin regeneration and wound healing, helping to maintain a youthful appearance. Humanin addresses cellular energy levels by protecting mitochondria, which are crucial for longevity. Epithalon helps to protect telomere length, which has been linked to aging and cellular decay.

Ideal For: Ideal for older adults looking to improve skin quality, reduce fatigue, and slow the aging process at the cellular level. It's also excellent for individuals looking for a holistic anti-aging approach that supports both external appearance and internal health.

How to Use: GHK-Cu is typically used topically or injected at 2-5 mg per dose. Humanin is taken subcutaneously at 100-200 mcg per dose, 2-3 times per week. Epithalon is given at 5-10 mg per dose for 10-20 days in a cycle. The combination should be cycled for 4-6 weeks, followed by a break.

---

4. Thymosin Beta-4 + Epithalon + Humanin: Tissue Regeneration and Cellular Health

Why Combine? Thymosin Beta-4 (TB-4) is a peptide that plays a crucial role in tissue repair and wound healing by promoting angiogenesis and cell migration. Boosting these processes helps in tissue regeneration, which is important for muscle recovery, joint health, and overall anti-aging. When combined with Epithalon, which works on telomere elongation and DNA repair, and Humanin, which supports mitochondrial health, this stack becomes a powerful tool for cellular regeneration and longevity.

Ideal For: Best suited for those who are looking to support cell regeneration, tissue repair, and longevity—particularly helpful for older adults suffering from joint degeneration, muscle loss, or chronic injuries. It's also beneficial for individuals wanting to improve mitochondrial function and prevent cellular aging.

How to Use TB-4 is injected subcutaneously at 2-5 mg per dose, 2-3 times per week. Epithalon is administered at 5-10 mg per dose for 10-20 days in a cycle. Humanin is taken subcutaneously at 100-200 mcg per dose, 2-3 times per week. This combination should be cycled for 4-6 weeks with breaks in between.

---

5. Follistatin 344 + Epithalon: Muscle Preservation and Cellular Health

Why Combine? Follistatin 344 is a peptide that inhibits myostatin, a protein that limits muscle growth. By blocking myostatin, it allows for increased muscle development, even as you age. Epithalon, by supporting telomere length, aids in slowing down the aging process, which is crucial for preserving muscle mass and cellular health in the long term. Together, these peptides work to promote muscle preservation, cellular rejuvenation, and overall longevity.

Ideal For: Ideal for older individuals or those who are concerned with muscle loss due to aging and who want to support longevity and cellular regeneration. It's especially useful for people who have experienced muscle wasting or those seeking a more youthful appearance and vitality.

How to Use: Follistatin 344 is injected subcutaneously at 0.5-1 mg per dose, 2-3 times a week. Epithalon is administered at 5-10 mg per dose for 10-20 days in a cycle. This combination should be cycled for 4-6 weeks, with breaks between cycles.

---

6. Humanin + Epithalon + GHK-Cu: Full-Body Rejuvenation

Why Combine? This powerful trio of peptides works on mitochondrial function (via Humanin), telomere protection (via Epithalon), and skin regeneration (via GHK-Cu), covering all the essential aspects of anti-aging. The combination works to support internal health by improving cellular energy production, while also preserving skin quality and structural integrity. It is a comprehensive approach to tackling aging from multiple angles.

Ideal For: Best for those who are looking for a well-rounded approach to aging, including older adults who are seeking to improve their cellular health, energy levels, skin condition, and overall longevity. This combination is ideal for those who want a holistic solution for aging.

How to Use Humanin is administered subcutaneously at 100-200 mcg per dose, 2-3 times per week. Epithalon is injected at 5-10 mg per dose for 10-20 days in cycles. GHK-Cu can be applied topically or injected at 2-5 mg per dose. This combination should be cycled for 4-6 weeks, followed by a break.

Peptides Combos for Immune Support

1-Thymosin Alpha-1 + BPC-157: Immune Function and Tissue Repair

Why Combine? Thymosin Alpha-1 (Tα1) is a peptide that boosts immune function by stimulating T-cell production and enhancing the body's defense against infections. It is particularly useful for immune system modulation and viral infections. BPC-157, while known for its wound healing properties, also has immune-boosting effects, particularly by reducing inflammation and aiding tissue repair, which is crucial when the body is recovering from an immune challenge.

Ideal For: Individuals looking to boost their immunity, especially those recovering from illness or chronic conditions where immune support and tissue repair are needed. It is also ideal for individuals who want to optimize immune function as they age.

How to Use: Thymosin Alpha-1 is typically administered subcutaneously at 1-2 mg per dose, 2-3 times a week. BPC-157 is used subcutaneously at 250 mcg per dose, 2-3 times a week. The combination can be cycled for 4-6 weeks, followed by a break.

2. Thymosin Beta-4 + Epithalon: Immune Health and Cellular Protection

Why Combine? Thymosin Beta-4 (TB-4) promotes tissue repair and immune regulation, particularly through its ability to enhance angiogenesis and reduce inflammation. It also aids in immune system modulation, enhancing overall cellular health. Epithalon works by protecting telomere length and maintaining cellular integrity, which is crucial for immune cell function as the body ages. Combining these two peptides helps both repair and protect immune cells while ensuring long-term immune health.

Ideal For: Those looking for a combination to help with immune system rejuvenation and cellular defense, especially for older adults or individuals with chronic inflammatory conditions or those exposed to stressors that challenge their immune system.

How to Use: Thymosin Beta-4 is administered subcutaneously at 2-5 mg per dose, 2-3 times a week. Epithalon is injected at 5-10 mg per dose for 10-20 days, followed by a rest period. This combination should be cycled for 4-6 weeks with a break between cycles.

3. Thymosin Alpha-1 + GHK-Cu + BPC-157: Immune Health and Tissue Regeneration

Why Combine? Thymosin Alpha-1 helps in stimulating T-cell activity and supports immune responses. GHK-Cu is a potent peptide that works by enhancing collagen production, promoting wound healing, and improving immune system health. It helps modulate the body's inflammatory response while supporting tissue regeneration. BPC-

157 supports inflammation control and wound healing, providing an additional boost to the immune system by enhancing tissue repair and reducing the time the body needs to recover from immune challenges.

Ideal For: This combination is perfect for individuals looking to boost immunity during illness recovery, chronic stress, or those looking to enhance tissue regeneration while promoting a strong immune system. It is particularly useful for athletes or individuals who are immunocompromised and need to support wound healing and immune function simultaneously.

How to Use: Thymosin Alpha-1 is administered subcutaneously at 1-2 mg per dose, 2-3 times a week. GHK-Cu can be applied topically or injected at 2-5 mg per dose. BPC-157 is injected at 250 mcg per dose, 2-3 times per week. This combination can be cycled for 4-6 weeks, followed by a rest phase.

---

4. Thymosin Alpha-1 + Humanin + Epithalon: Immune and Mitochondrial Support

Why Combine? Thymosin Alpha-1 boosts the body's immune response by promoting T-cell function and immune regulation, while Humanin works on improving mitochondrial function, which is essential for overall cellular health and energy production. Epithalon helps extend telomeres, promoting long-term cellular health and enhancing immune function as the body ages. This powerful trio works together to ensure immune system health and cellular longevity.

Ideal For: Individuals interested in long-term immune health and mitochondrial support, particularly useful for older individuals, chronic illness recovery, or anyone experiencing fatigue or immune challenges due to aging or lifestyle factors.

How to Use: Thymosin Alpha-1 is taken subcutaneously at 1-2 mg per dose, 2-3 times a week. Humanin is typically injected subcutaneously at 100-200 mcg per dose, 2-3 times a week. Epithalon is injected at 5-10 mg per dose for 10-20 days in cycles. This combination can be used for 4-6 weeks, followed by a break.

---

5. BPC-157 + GHK-Cu + Thymosin Beta-4: Immune Modulation and Healing

Why Combine? BPC-157 is an anti-inflammatory peptide that supports the repair of tissues and promotes immune modulation. GHK-Cu is essential for immune health, promoting collagen synthesis and enhancing wound healing, while also acting as a powerful anti-inflammatory agent. Thymosin Beta-4 boosts immune responses and supports the healing of tissues through angiogenesis, making this combination ideal for those who need to boost immune resilience and enhance tissue regeneration at the same time.

Ideal For: Best suited for individuals recovering from injury or chronic conditions that impair the immune system and tissue repair. Also beneficial for anyone looking to boost immunity and reduce inflammation in the body, particularly in cases of autoimmune disorders or immune system imbalance.

How to Use: B PC-157 is administered subcutaneously at 250 mcg per dose, 2-3 times per week. GHK-Cu is applied topically or injected at 2-5 mg per dose, and Thymosin Beta-4 is injected subcutaneously at 2-5 mg per dose, 2-3 times per week. This combination can be used for 4-6 weeks, followed by a rest phase.

---

6. Thymosin Alpha-1 + Humanin + BPC-157: Immune Support and Regeneration

Why Combine? Thymosin Alpha-1 strengthens the immune system by enhancing T-cell production and supporting immune modulation. Humanin focuses on mitochondrial health, which is crucial for maintaining energy levels and cellular function, indirectly supporting the immune system's ability to function optimally. BPC-157 promotes tissue repair and reduces inflammation, which is beneficial during recovery from illness or immune challenges.

Ideal For: Suitable for individuals looking to boost immune function and promote tissue regeneration after illness, injury, or stress. It is especially beneficial for those looking for long-term immunity support and cellular rejuvenation.

How to Use: Thymosin Alpha-1 is injected subcutaneously at 1-2 mg per dose, 2-3 times per week. Humanin is injected at 100-200 mcg per dose, 2-3 times a week. BPC-157 is used at 250 mcg per dose, 2-3 times a week. This combination should be cycled for 4-6 weeks, with breaks in between.

Peptides Combos for Hormones Health

1. Kisspeptin-10 + PT-141: Libido and Hormonal Balance

Why Combine? Kisspeptin-10 is a key peptide involved in reproductive hormone regulation, particularly in stimulating the release of GnRH (gonadotropin-releasing hormone), which triggers the production of LH (luteinizing hormone) and FSH (follicle-stimulating hormone), hormones responsible for sexual function and fertility. PT-141 (Bremelanotide), on the other hand, acts directly on the brain's melanocortin receptors to improve libido and sexual arousal by stimulating the dopamine system. Together, they offer a powerful combination for enhancing sexual desire and restoring hormonal balance, making them particularly effective for those experiencing low libido or hormonal imbalances.

Ideal For: Men and women experiencing low libido or sexual dysfunction due to age, hormonal changes, or stress. It is also suitable for those undergoing hormonal therapy or dealing with the effects of chronic illness on sexual health.

How to Use: Kisspeptin-10 is typically administered subcutaneously at a dose of 0.5-1 mg, 1-2 times a week. PT-141 is injected subcutaneously at 1-2 mg per dose as needed, typically before sexual activity. The combination can be cycled for 4-6 weeks, followed by a break to assess effectiveness.

2. Melanotan II + Kisspeptin-10: Sexual Health and Hormonal Regulation

Why Combine? Melanotan II has been shown to increase sexual arousal and libido through its action on melanocortin receptors, similar to PT-141, but with the added benefit of also stimulating melanin production, which helps to darken the skin. This peptide is often used to treat sexual dysfunction and enhance sexual desire. When combined with Kisspeptin-10, which influences the reproductive hormone axis and the release of GnRH, this combination can improve both the hormonal balance and sexual function.

Ideal For: This combination is beneficial for both men and women experiencing sexual dysfunction, especially those with hormonal imbalances due to aging or medical treatments. It is also suitable for individuals seeking to improve sexual health without the use of invasive treatments.

How to Use: Melanotan II is administered subcutaneously at 0.5-1 mg per dose, 3-4 times a week, while Kisspeptin-10 is used at 0.5-1 mg per dose, 1-2 times per week. This combination can be cycled for 4-6 weeks, with a break in between to assess efficacy.

3. PT-141 + Growth Hormone Secretagogues (GHRP-6): Sexual Health and Growth Hormone Stimulation

Why Combine? PT-141 (Bremelanotide) directly boosts sexual arousal and libido, working through the melanocortin receptors to improve sexual function. Growth Hormone Secretagogues like GHRP-6 stimulate the pituitary gland to release growth hormone, which plays a critical role in muscle recovery, fat metabolism, and sexual health. The combination of these two peptides promotes not only enhanced sexual desire but also overall hormonal health by stimulating both growth hormone production and sexual function.

Ideal For: This combination is perfect for individuals seeking to enhance their sexual health while simultaneously improving overall vitality. It's ideal for men and women over 40 experiencing hormonal decline, those recovering from chronic illness, or athletes looking for better recovery and sexual health.

How to Use: PT-141 is used subcutaneously at a dose of 1-2 mg, as needed before sexual activity, while GHRP-6 is taken subcutaneously at 100-200 mcg, 2-3 times per week. The combination should be cycled for 4-6 weeks, followed by a rest period.

4. Kisspeptin-10 + GHRH + PT-141: Comprehensive Sexual Health and Hormonal Optimization

Why Combine? Kisspeptin-10 triggers the release of GnRH, stimulating LH and FSH, which are crucial for reproductive function. GHRH (Growth Hormone-Releasing Hormone) works by stimulating the pituitary gland to secrete growth hormone, which enhances muscle mass, fat metabolism, and sexual health. Together, these peptides work synergistically to support hormonal balance, sexual function, and overall vitality, while PT-141 increases sexual desire and arousal by activating the brain's melanocortin receptors.

Ideal For: Ideal for both men and women dealing with age-related hormone decline or those seeking to optimize their sexual health and general vitality. It's particularly useful for those with low libido, muscle loss, or fat accumulation due to hormonal changes.

How to Use: Kisspeptin-10 is taken subcutaneously at 0.5-1 mg per dose, 1-2 times per week. GHRH is injected at 100-200 mcg 2-3 times a week, while PT-141 is administered subcutaneously at 1-2 mg before sexual activity. This combination should be cycled for 4-6 weeks.

5. Melanotan II + CJC-1295 + Ipamorelin: Libido and Growth Hormone Boost

Why Combine? Melanotan II improves libido and sexual arousal via the melanocortin receptors while also promoting melanin production. CJC-1295 is a growth hormone-releasing hormone (GHRH) analog that stimulates the release of growth hormone, supporting muscle growth, fat loss, and sexual vitality. Ipamorelin is a growth hormone secretagogue that helps increase growth hormone levels without raising prolactin levels, enhancing both muscle building and sexual health. This combination supports sexual function while promoting muscle recovery, fat loss, and overall rejuvenation.

Ideal For: Best for individuals looking to improve sexual health while enhancing muscle mass and fat metabolism. It's ideal for men over 40, individuals suffering from hormonal imbalances, or athletes seeking to optimize both sexual health and muscle recovery.

How to Use: Melanotan II is used subcutaneously at 0.5-1 mg, 3-4 times per week. CJC-1295 and Ipamorelin are both injected subcutaneously at 100-200 mcg per dose, 2-3 times a week. This combination can be cycled for 4-6 weeks, followed by a break.

---

6. Kisspeptin-10 + Epithalon + PT-141: Hormonal Health, Sexual Function, and Longevity

Why Combine? Kisspeptin-10 helps regulate GnRH release, which is crucial for sexual function and hormonal balance. Epithalon is a telomerase activator that supports cellular health and promotes longevity by extending telomere length. PT-141 stimulates sexual arousal and desire by working on the brain's melanocortin receptors. Together, this trio works on improving hormonal balance, supporting sexual health, and promoting longevity by protecting cellular integrity.

Ideal For: Suitable for those looking to support their sexual health, hormonal balance, and overall well-being while seeking longevity benefits. This is ideal for both men and women dealing with aging-related sexual dysfunction or those wanting to maintain youthful vitality.

How to Use: Kisspeptin-10 is injected subcutaneously at 0.5-1 mg 1-2 times per week. Epithalon is administered subcutaneously at 5-10 mg for 10-20 days in cycles. PT-141 is used as needed, subcutaneously at 1-2 mg before sexual activity.

CONCLUSIONS

The therapeutic potential of peptides is a rapidly expanding research area. Between 2016 and 2022, the FDA approved 26 peptide-based drugs out of more than 315 new drug approvals, with over 200 peptides in clinical trials and 600 more in preclinical phases. The rise in scientific publications and patents highlights the expanding focus on peptides. These compounds are in development for diverse treatments, such as microbial infections, obesity, and cancer, and are also being used to advance cell-targeting and cell-penetrating technologies.

Notably, cell-penetrating peptides are being explored as delivery tools for anti-cancer, antibacterial, and antiviral therapies.

However, as the field advances, the need for sustainable synthesis practices has become equally pressing. As peptide research and production grow, so does the demand for greener, more efficient methods. Techniques such as water-based SPPS, LPPS, and microwave-assisted synthesis offer promising steps toward eco-friendly solutions. Yet, more progress remains to be made to meet both the scientific and ethical challenges in peptide production.

Embracing these technologies, academic researchers and the pharmaceutical industry are poised to drive peptide science forward in a sustainable direction, fostering the next wave of innovation that balances efficacy with environmental responsibility. This journey toward sustainable and accessible peptide therapies signals modern medicine's exciting and impactful future.